Praise for
The Diet-Free Revolution

"With engaging storytelling and insightful analysis, Alexis Conason offers a truly weight-inclusive approach to mindful eating that will help you develop self-compassion, practice self-care, and find pleasure in food and your body."

—CHRISTY HARRISON, MPH, RD, author of
Anti-Diet

"I absolutely love this brilliant book from Dr. Conason. Smart, compassionate, with relatable and vivid stories and specific practice recommendations throughout, *The Diet-Free Revolution* embodies the most cutting-edge blend of science and psychology while acknowledging vital social justice themes. I am delighted to have this book as a resource that I will recommend to my patients and their families as well as to anyone seeking to transform their relationship with their body and food."

—JENNIFER L. GAUDIANI, MD, CEDS-S, FAED,
founder and medical director of the Gaudiani Clinic
and author of *Sick Enough*

"This book is *truly* a revolution and a chance to break free from the tyranny of diets and food obsession for good. Alexis Conason is an expert on the subject and understands how layered this journey can be. There are deep cultural and psychological factors that keep us clinging to diets, and this book leaves no stone unturned."

—CAROLINE DOONER, author of *The F*ck It Diet*

"You have what it takes to heal your relationship with food. Dr. Conason's simple 10-step plan will encourage you to be kind to yourself while bravely leaving behind the misery of dieting once and for all!"

—REBECCA SCRITCHFIELD, RDN, EP-C, author

"In my work as a journalist, I talk to people every day who are starting to recognize that years of dieting have sabotaged their relationships with food and their bodies—but they don't know what else to do or how to stop. It is such a relief to be able to point them to *The Diet-Free Revolution*, which provides a clear, empathetic, and evidence-based roadmap for the work and healing that comes next. Conason is the warm, wise therapist and friend you've been looking for. And her certainty that radical self-acceptance and food freedom are possible for anyone will put these concepts within reach of those struggling the most."

—VIRGINIA SOLE-SMITH, author of *The Eating Instinct*

"The most important thing I have to say about Alexis Conason's book is that it is supremely trustworthy. With an exquisite balance of research, personal and professional insights, mindfulness expertise, and understanding of intersectional social justice issues, this book is the one you need to heal your relationship with food and your precious body. *Vive la révolution!*"

—JENNA HOLLENSTEIN, MS, RDN, CDN, author of *Eat to Love*

"Written with compassion, wisdom, and a touch of humor, *The Diet-Free Revolution* will give you the skills and strategies you need to create a peaceful and nurturing relationship with food."

—JUDITH MATZ, coauthor of *The Body Positivity Card Deck* and *The Diet Survivor's Handbook*

"The ultimate guide to why diets don't work and what to do instead—backed by strong and plentiful science. . . . This book is a must-read for both professionals and the general public who are seeking to end the suffering and embrace the joy of eating and living."

—LYNN ROSSY, PhD, author of *Savor Every Bite*

"Lovingly written, but backed by the best modern science, *The Diet-Free Revolution* lights a clear path, step by step, toward an emotional freedom that most dieters have long ago given up hope of achieving."

—STEPHEN SNYDER, MD, associate clinical professor at the Icahn School of Medicine at Mount Sinai and author of *Love Worth Making*

"In a world that teaches us to devote our entire lives to the pursuit of thinness, this book is a reminder that it's possible to break free from the diet cycle and live our damn lives. This book is like one big, warm therapy session with enough science and practical skills to make an anti-diet life an actual reality. We all need this book in our lives."

—SHIRA ROSENBLUTH, LCSW, eating
disorder therapist, activist, and founder of
www.theshirarose.com

"If you are ready to stop punishing yourself with endless cycles of starvation diets followed by out-of-control eating, negative self-talk, and feelings of failure, *The Diet-Free Revolution* offers a wonderful and practical road map forward. Dr. Alexis Conason weaves stories and real-life examples—all supported by science— that will show you what you truly need to thrive."

—ERICA LEON, MS, RDN, CDN, CEDRD, reg-
istered dietitian, certified eating disorders registered
dietitian, certified intuitive eating counselor, and
owner of Erica Leon Nutrition LLC

"Not only does Dr. Alexis Conason give you the 'why' you shouldn't diet, she gives you specific action steps on what to do instead to create a healthy relationship with food. Her advice is thoughtful, realistic, and appropriate for anyone who has had a chronic up-and-down journey with dieting."

—JENNIFER MCGURK, RDN, CDN, CEDRD-S,
certified eating disorders registered dietitian and
clinical supervisor and owner of Pursuing Private
Practice

"*The Diet-Free Revolution* is about finding a sustainable, realistic path to overall health—at any size. By combatting the root causes of disordered eating and body image with mindfulness and therapy, we can finally begin to heal and be free to live our lives fully, peacefully, and healthily."

—RENEE CAFARO, US editor of *SLiNK* magazine
and plus-size influencer

The
Diet-Free
Revolution

The
Diet-Free
Revolution

10 Steps to Free Yourself from the Diet Cycle with Mindful Eating and Radical Self-Acceptance

ALEXIS CONASON, PsyD

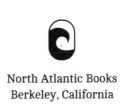

North Atlantic Books
Berkeley, California

Published by
North Atlantic Books
Berkeley, California

Cover photo © Ruth Black/Shutterstock.com
Cover design by Jess Morphew
Book design by Happenstance Type-O-Rama

Printed in Canada

The Diet-Free Revolution: 10 Steps to Free Yourself from the Diet Cycle with Mindful Eating and Radical Self-Acceptance is sponsored and published by North Atlantic Books, an educational nonprofit based in Berkeley, California, that collaborates with partners to develop cross-cultural perspectives, nurture holistic views of art, science, the humanities, and healing, and seed personal and global transformation by publishing work on the relationship of body, spirit, and nature.

North Atlantic Books' publications are distributed to the US trade and internationally by Penguin Random House Publishers Services. For further information, visit our website at www.northatlanticbooks.com

MEDICAL DISCLAIMER: The following information is intended for general information purposes only. Individuals should always see their health care provider before administering any suggestions made in this book. Any application of the material set forth in the following pages is at the reader's discretion and is their sole responsibility.

Library of Congress Cataloging-in-Publication Data
Names: Conason, Alexis, author.
Title: The diet-free revolution : 10 steps to free yourself from the diet
   cycle with mindful eating and radical self-acceptance / Alexis Conason.
Description: Berkeley, CA : North Atlantic Books, [2021] | Includes
   bibliographical references and index. | Summary: "A guide for leaving
   diet culture and healing your relationship with food"—Provided by
   publisher.
Identifiers: LCCN 2020053833 | ISBN 9781623176198 (trade paperback) | ISBN
   9781623176204 (ebook)
Subjects: LCSH: Self-acceptance. | Food habits—Psychological aspects. |
   Food—Psychological aspects. | Diet—Psychological aspects.
Classification: LCC BF575.S37 C66 2021 | DDC 158.1—dc23
LC record available at https://lccn.loc.gov/2020053833

1 2 3 4 5 6 7 8 9 MARQUIS 26 25 24 23 22 21

This book includes recycled material and material from well-managed forests. North Atlantic Books is committed to the protection of our environment. We print on recycled paper whenever possible and partner with printers who strive to use environmentally responsible practices.

For Roberta and Emilia,
May you always know that you are
good enough, exactly as you are

Contents

Introduction

If you're like most people, you've spent a lot of your life thinking about what to eat. And what not to eat. And feeling like crap about your body.

You've done what any rational person would do—you tried to change your body by dieting. Again … and again … and yet again. Each time you started a new diet, you were filled with hope and yearning—*finally, I'm going to get the life I've always wanted! More energy! Better health! Respect! Sex appeal!* But it was only a matter of time before you fell off the wagon and that optimism was replaced by shame and self-blame—*how could I have failed at this again?* You berated yourself as you ate a pint of ice cream, standing in the kitchen with the freezer still open. Or perhaps it was the tsunami of guilt after ordering the pasta with cream sauce when you had promised yourself you would "be good" and get the chicken breast. Each time you strayed away from the prescribed methods of another plan, you vowed to be better, to get back on track, and you once again doubled down on the dieting game.

I get it. I've been there too. I spent most of my life on and off diet plans. I went on my first juice cleanse when I was eight years old. I found the instructions in one of the countless diet books that lined the bookshelves of my family's living room. My mother was a chronic dieter, and I learned early on that dieting and overeating was the way of life. Big appetites were our family hallmark and dieting was how we combated it. When we went out to eat, the menu was always a focal point of discussion. "If I were going to cheat today, I would certainly get the pasta with seafood," my mother would say salaciously. "Or maybe the ribs?" my father would suggest before both would order the grilled fish, politely asking the waiter if it would be possible to substitute the roasted potatoes that came on the side for some steamed spinach and go light on the oil, please.

While my mother rarely commented on my body directly, the scorn for her own body spoke louder than words. Bodies were objects to be wrestled into submission. Food was a substance to exert control over or to surrender yourself to. As a child, I discovered that eating helped me cope with my internal struggles. Food was my companion, a source of comfort and pleasure in bleak moments. But as adolescence brought unwanted curves and unsolicited attention, food also became the enemy. My body took the blame for my unhappiness, and I was convinced that, if I could just get my body to conform, I could finally have the love and acceptance I craved. I found myself caught in a vicious cycle. The more I dieted, the more out of control I felt around food. The more I ate, the more I hated my body. And the more I despised my body, the more convinced I became that dieting was the answer. For nearly two decades, around and around I went.

Even though I was failing at dieting—or more accurately, dieting was failing me—I was committed to the weight loss paradigm. It was such an ingrained part of my life that I never questioned it. After all, it wasn't just me who was dieting. Everyone around me was doing it too. My friend would call me in a panic after having eaten a sandwich, desperately asking for reassurance that two pieces of bread wouldn't make her gain weight. When we went out to dinner, salads (dressing on the side, please!) were the norm. Stopping for "ice cream" clearly meant fat-free Froyo. One of my friends used the phrase "she looked so anorexic" as a compliment (for the record, anorexia is a serious mental illness). At the time, the only thing that seemed abnormal in all of this was my craving for french fries and chow fun noodles.

After college, I decided to pursue a career in psychology with the intention of helping other people lose weight. Because when you can't figure out your own stuff, of course you'll be a pro at figuring out everyone else's!

I spent five years in graduate school learning psychological strategies to help people eat less and exercise more, did postdoctoral work in "obesity" research, trained at a bariatric weight loss surgery clinic, and eventually hung up my shingle proclaiming that I was open for business as a psychologist specializing in weight management.

That's when reality smacked me in the face: The strategies I learned in school didn't work! Just like dieting didn't work for me, it didn't work for my clients. In fact, the harder my clients tried to control their eating, the more out of control they spiraled. They were stuck in the same cycle I was in. And it wasn't just us. At "obesity" research conferences, I heard study after study presented with dismal results detailing the different ways people failed to lose weight and keep it off long-term. It was clear that experts had no idea how to help people lose significant weight in a sustainable way.

In a panic about the bleak outlook of my newly minted career, I began to search for something different. I discovered mindful eating and learned about weight-inclusive approaches to health. I embraced the radical notions that my value is not determined by my body size or my health and that I deserved a life full of respect, love, and pleasure regardless of what size pants I was wearing. Bodies naturally exist across a diverse spectrum of shapes and sizes, and this is a fact to admire, not admonish. My eating started to feel more in control once I stopped trying so frantically to control it; but more importantly I stopped thinking about food all the time, and the deep shame I had carried since childhood started to ease.

And this is what I want to share with you, that it is possible to feel better about your eating and body—but not in the ways that most of us have been taught.

I spent the next ten years of my career developing The Anti-Diet Plan program, a unique blend of psychological, mindfulness, and cultural-change strategies to help you get unstuck from old patterns of dieting and learn a radically new way of eating and relating to the world. What started as a small group that met in my Manhattan office is now an online program available worldwide. I have helped hundreds of people break free from the diet–binge–self-hatred cycle. Even people who struggled for decades have learned to fundamentally change their eating behaviors in a sustainable way. My clients learned to turn down the volume on their destructive self-talk, reconnect with their appetite in an aware and trusting way, and develop a nonjudgmental, accepting, and compassionate relationship with their body. They have opened their eyes to the oppressive systems that convince us our bodies are flawed, and chosen a path toward body liberation instead of dieting. It's amazing what can happen when we heal our relationship with food and body! Instead of living our life trying to be as small as possible, we can take up the space that we deserve in the world. Now it's your turn.

Welcome to *The Diet-Free Revolution*. If you've had enough of failed diets and feeling like a failure, get ready to learn a new way of eating and relating to food. Eating does not need to be a struggle. This book will help you find a peaceful and nurturing relationship with food. Consider this your ticket off the dieting roller coaster filled with peaks of restrictive eating, plummeting descents into out-of-control eating, and stomach-churning loop de loops of failure and self-hatred. If you want to be free from conflicts with eating, be more content with your body, and have more mental space for the things that matter most in your life, this book is for you.

Why Be Diet-Free?

For many of us, dieting is like a bad relationship. We just can't seem to stay away, even though the cycle exhausts us. For anyone who has ever been in an unhealthy relationship—whether it's a toxic friendship, a controlling romantic partner, or a narcissistic boss—you may relate to the feeling of being pulled in by something dark that makes you feel good and bad at the same time. We get so entranced by the fantasy of what *could be* that we overlook the reality of *what is*.

When I was younger, I was particularly drawn to these kinds of relationships. For years I dated someone who was emotionally abusive. He ran hot and cold, became enraged at the slightest perceived offense, and seemed to take pleasure in tearing me down. I held him up on a pedestal, believing that if I could earn his good favor I would finally find relief from the pain that welled up inside of me. My world narrowed until he was the only thing in it—earning his affection was my singular life goal. For the most part, he was critical and demeaning toward me. But on the rare occasions when I was in his good graces, it was like being fed nectar from the gods. I savored the sweet drops and tried to sustain myself on them, though they were few and far between. I believed that one day, if I could just figure out how to be good enough, I would earn a steady stream of nectar. It took me a long time to figure out that the stream didn't exist; the tiny droplets were all he had to offer.

How many of us are sustaining ourselves on the droplets of nectar offered by diets? That time when you stuck to the plan, the moment when you got to your goal weight, that evening when you felt on top of the world? Those are the droplets, the sweet tastes of all that dieting promises us. It's these drops that keep us holding on during all the bad stuff—through the shame, the self-hatred, the loss of control, the feelings of failure—and believing that if we can just get it right, we'll tap into an endless stream of nectar. Spoiler alert: diets have no more than droplets to give. The rest is just a mirage.

Despite our personal experiences with diet after diet (or "lifestyle change" after "lifestyle change") that failed to result in long-term weight loss, we remain convinced that this time will be different. *This time, the diet will work and provide me with all that I'm looking for.* We are brainwashed into believing that diets are the answer and *we* are the problem. Rather than celebrating the natural diversity of body shapes and sizes, the diet-industrial complex convinces us that any deviations from the designated ideal body are moral shortcomings that must be extinguished with proper discipline and righteousness. Inability to conform to this ideal through dieting is a sign of moral inferiority. In one of the most successful hoaxes of modern times, the weight loss industry has convinced us that it is *our* fault their products have failed. Shifting the spotlight to capitalize on our own insecurities rather than the failures of the diet plans keeps us dependent on the very industry that harms us. If the popular plans really worked, we would go on one (not hundreds), lose weight, maintain the weight loss, and be able to stay on the plan for its duration. Diets would be a one-time investment. Instead we enroll over and over again, spending our valuable time, emotional energy, and money on products that are inherently flawed. We are taught—and then tell ourselves—that we can't stick to our diets because we are weak-willed, lazy, and gluttonous. We beat ourselves up for our perceived failures and set out in search of the only thing that will make us feel better: another diet! And there is always another diet waiting for us with the promise of a thinner, healthier, happier, and better life.

What would you do if your hairdresser gave you a terrible haircut and then told you that the problem was your hair? Would you keep buying clothes that fell apart days after the first time you wore them? What if, when you tried to return them, you were told that it's your fault the clothes ripped because you wore them wrong? Would you eat at a restaurant where the food tasted spoiled, and when you complained to the waiter, you were told that the food is fine, the problem is your taste buds? In other areas of our life, if a product is faulty we stop using it. We may even ask for our money back or write a negative review online to warn others. Why is dieting so different? Why are we so convinced that we need diets even after all our personal experiences tell us loud and clear that they don't work?

The program formerly known as Weight Watchers, now renamed WW, is a great example of how dieting creates a culture of dependency that profits off its failures. WW confers a coveted free "lifetime membership" status to members who have reached their goal weight and maintained it for more than six weeks. After being bestowed this "honor," lifetime members must attend WW meetings and weigh in every single month. If you miss a month or go more than two pounds above your goal weight, *ka-ching!*, WW cashes in and you start paying the monthly fee again.[1] This creates a cult-like dependency in which members are indoctrinated into the program week after week, often for years or decades, lest they lose their lifetime status. When members inevitably gain weight, they are punished (by needing to pay again) and the program is seen as the savior (if they recommit, start paying for meetings again, and get back down to their goal weight, they can earn back their status). This strategy of repeat business led to WW raking in $1.4 billion in 2019—and that was one of the company's less profitable years![2]

Nearly half of all adults in the US try to lose weight each year.[3] In 2012, 108 million people went on a diet, and in 2019 people spent $72 billion in pursuit of weight loss.[4] The wellness industry, dieting's close cousin, is valued at $4.5 trillion globally.[5] The average dieter attempts four to five diets per year because success eludes them.[6] One survey found that the average adult tries 126 diets over the course of their life and stays on each one for about six days.[7] Does this mean that we are all failures? Or have diets failed us? These numbers underscore the primary problem with dieting: diets are designed to fail. They keep us stuck in the belief that our bodies are the problem instead of challenging the cultural forces invested in our believing that lie.

Diets are more than benignly ineffective; they can be downright harmful. As we'll learn about in chapter 1, incessant cycles of being on and off a diet wreak havoc on our physical and mental well-being. Dieting is associated with increased risk of eating disorders and disordered eating, body image dissatisfaction, weight cycling (or the weight loss–weight gain roller coaster), internalized weight bias (i.e., the way that we take our negative stereotypes about fat people and turn them inward toward ourselves), metabolic disease (including diabetes), earlier death, and more.

Not only do diets cause suffering on a personal level, they also cause systemic social harm. Dieting is part of "diet culture," a widespread system of beliefs that equates thinness and weight loss with health, moral value, desirability, and superiority. Diet culture is an amalgamation of systems of oppression, including (but not limited to) the patriarchy, capitalism, and white supremacy. (If the connections between dieting and these systems of oppression don't immediately seem clear, don't worry, we'll be unpacking it all as we go through the program). In her book *The Beauty Myth*, author Naomi Wolf says: "A culture fixated on female thinness is not an obsession about female beauty, but an obsession about female obedience."[8] Diet culture distracts us from social and political action. It occupies precious emotional energy, exhausts us, and makes it difficult to engage fully in other areas of our life. It obscures our vision and makes it hard to clearly see what is happening around us. For example, when we are consumed with thoughts about how many calories are in our scone, we aren't thinking about why white women are paid 15 percent less than white men, or why Black women are paid 38 percent less than white men and 21 percent less than white women.[9] When we are googling whether multigrain or spelt bread is "healthier," we aren't looking up why one in nine people in the US don't have enough to eat.[10] When we are hiding in the back of the room because we don't want people to see our body, we don't get up to the mic to have our voice heard. Dieting is a tool of an oppressive system invested in keeping us focused on changing our bodies instead of changing the world. When I talk about diet culture in this book, please keep in mind that I'm talking about not just the act of dieting but also the systems of oppression that are inextricably linked.

Women have been disproportionately affected by the demands of dieting. Studies suggest that over 90 percent of women are dissatisfied with their body and want to lose weight. In contrast, about 40 percent of men report dissatisfaction with their body.[11] Clearly, both women and men struggle with body image issues, but women are hit far harder. Transgender folks and, to a lesser extent, gay men also struggle with higher rates of body image dissatisfaction than cisgender heterosexual men. Unlike men, who tend to be valued for wealth and power, women are valued for appearance. When women don't conform to the Eurocentric thin ideal of beauty and health, they lose their social capital. In a world where women are already second-rate citizens, weight loss is seen as a fast track to increasing status. Later in this book, we will also learn how the pursuit of thinness can be traced back to racist origins. Unfortunately, the reality is that dieting keeps us confined to the very same powerless positions we seek to escape.

From the "war on obesity" to the celebrities we admire to the way that we are treated at our doctors' offices, there is no mistaking that the most desirable body type is thin. We turn on the television, pick up a magazine, or scroll through social media and seldom see people who look like us—instead we see an unachievable thin ideal. This is especially true for Black,

Indigenous, and People of Color (BIPOC) populations, trans and nonbinary people, fat people (see "A Note on Language and Identity" at the end of this chapter for a discussion on the term *fat*), people with disabilities, and those with other marginalized identities who almost never see themselves represented in desirable ways. We are confronted with images of what we should, and (for some of us) perhaps even *could*, look like if only we had the proper discipline. We rarely see images affirming our current body.

While there are certain universalities to struggles with food and body image, these struggles are heightened for people living in marginalized bodies who are pushed to the sidelines of society and denied access to power and resources, compared with those living in bodies deemed socially acceptable. It is exponentially harder to accept your body when your body is demonized by the world around you. If you are living in a larger body, you are likely confronted on a daily basis with the fact that the world was not designed for your body. Each time a clothing store doesn't carry your size, or you wonder if you can slide into the narrow banquette at a restaurant, or you are forced to pay for two seats on an airplane, or someone gives you a side-eye when you go to sit next to them, you are implicitly being told that your body doesn't belong. When you get passed over for a job promotion, get rejected on a dating app, or have your health complaints ignored by your doctor, you are forced to decipher whether or not this is happening because of your body size. Accepting your body becomes even more challenging for those with multiple marginalized identities that layer over each other and intersect in different ways. For example, fat Black women are forced to contend with fatphobia and racism and sexism. Fat Black queer women must deal with fatphobia, racism, sexism, and homophobia. The world was designed for thin straight white bodies, and the further that you deviate from that "norm" the more societal hostility you will face and the more messages you will receive telling you that your body is bad.

This is hard to contend with. It's important to remember that the problem is *not* your body. The problem is diet culture.

Diet culture fosters pervasive mistrust in our bodies and ubiquitous conflicts around food. We are caught in a cultural mass delusion that weight loss is a feasible path to alleviating our suffering. We are taught that fat bodies are just containers for thin ones waiting to emerge. Based on a calculation of height and weight called the body mass index (BMI, or the bullshit measuring index, as I like to call it), doctors issue reprimands for presumed poor health, warning of the risk of diabetes, high blood pressure, heart disease, and cancer—all without ever drawing a single vial of blood. Diet recommendations are doled out liberally, as if the only thing standing between a fat person and the thinner person they should become is the novel idea to eat less and exercise more.

Even though dieting fails most people, stories of dieting success abound, making success seem like the norm. Our coworker who is two weeks into intermittent fasting can say confidently that it works. "It's not a diet! It's a way of life!" they proclaim. Your friend who started eliminating sugar last week already feels so much better. And have you seen how much weight Oprah lost on WW? She can eat bread! A lot of attention is given to the vocal minority of people who experience weight loss success, even when that success comes in the early "honeymoon" phase of dieting—which is almost always followed by predictable weight regain—or when the success story is the exception to the norm (i.e., the roughly 5 percent of people who are able to sustain weight loss long-term, sometimes through eating-disordered behaviors, surgery, or medications). Ever notice how the before and after pictures in diet advertisements specify "results not typical?" The spotlight on dieting success stories (and quiet around subsequent weight regain) makes it seem like diets work for everyone but us. Why can't we have the same success? What's wrong with us? We conclude that the problem must be us, not the diet. This way of thinking fosters mistrust in ourselves and keeps us going back to diets again and again.

Our society is in the midst of an epidemic of disordered eating. We are tossed around like a ping-pong ball: on the wagon, off the wagon, restricting and dieting, feeling out of control, consumed with thoughts of food, hating our bodies. It is all normalized; we are even praised when our efforts lead to weight loss (followed by eerie silence or snide remarks when the weight inevitably comes back on). We look to others to tell us what we should and shouldn't eat. We turn our friends and family into diet enforcers, desperately pleading, "Please don't let me eat that dessert!" and "Don't you dare bring those chips into the house!" Doctors, both those who treat us and those we see in the media, are the diet dictators, instructing us to eat this and not that. Instagram celebrities are our most trusted sources of nutritional guidance. We become infantilized—unable to trust that we know what we really need. But this is not true! Just like Dorothy trying to find her way home from Oz, we have the power within us. We hold an intrinsic knowledge of how to truly care for and nurture ourselves.

The Revolution Is Ready for You

The Diet-Free Revolution is not a quick fix. It involves forgiving ourselves, reconnecting with our bodies, and relearning how to feed and nurture ourselves at the most basic level. It encourages us to direct our anger toward diet culture, where it belongs, rather than taking aim at our own body. It teaches us how to use principles of mindfulness meditation to listen to the inherent wisdom of our body to guide our eating in a radically new way. Above all, it's about regaining a sense of trust in ourselves. The answer to your problems does not lie within the next diet plan. The answer is within **you**. This book will help you learn how to tune in to your internal well of knowledge, turn up the volume on your "internal GPS" navigation system, and hear your body again. It will support you in the profound learning that "nothing tastes better than being thin feels" is the marketing lie that keeps people bound to diets and cycles of disordered eating. It prevents us from achieving the rich, full, authentic life we deserve at any size.

The Diet-Free Revolution has no dietary restrictions and no pill or supplement requirements. You will not cleanse or detoxify your body (your body does a great job of that all on its own—thank you, liver!). This program does not come with appetite-suppressing teas that promise to give you a belly like the stars. You don't need to run out and stock your pantry with special diet foods or buy any new scales, counters, or trackers. The best part is, you already have everything you need!

The basic tenet of *The Diet-Free Revolution* is that eating is informed from within. It is premised on the radical idea that your body is inherently good—even when it struggles—and, with nurturance, care, and communication, it can lead you on the path toward well-being. This may be hard to believe, but trust me, even if you think your body is untrustworthy or uncooperative, it is possible! When you are fully present and aware, without judgment, you can clearly hear the innate signals your body is sending you. In the following chapters, I'll be walking you through how to do all of this. You will relearn how to feed and nourish your unique miraculous body. This practice encourages more satisfaction and pleasure when eating, less preoccupation and conflict around food, including choosing foods that make your body feel good, reduced stress, and overall improved mental and physical health.

Ultimately, *The Diet-Free Revolution* is not just about changing the way you relate to food; it's about changing the way you relate to yourself and achieving your own optimal health. In this book, I use the term *health* to mean your own definition of well-being; it's not an external definition of health or a medical definition of health but a general sense of feeling *your* best in *your* body, even if your body isn't doing exactly what you want it to do. The strategies in this book are designed to foster a kinder, gentler, and more compassionate way of being. Too many of us live with a harsh inner voice that criticizes us day in and day out. We believe that this "tough love" will motivate us to change, but that couldn't be further from the truth. In fact, it's this very voice that is keeping us stuck. Change occurs from a place of self-love, not self-hatred. When we believe that our bodies are bad, we carry a deep sense of shame and failure. We retreat from the world. In trying to make our bodies small, we make our lives small. The truth is, our bodies, in all their various forms and despite the different challenges they may face, are doing the best that they can. After all, they keep us alive and that is pretty damn incredible. My hope is that you will come to see your body as incredible, even if you don't always like your body, even if you wish it was different, even if it doesn't work the way you want or need it to, and even if you live in a body that the world doesn't approve of. Because hating a body is exhausting. It keeps us stuck and prevents us from living our best lives. You deserve a life full of meaning, pleasure, and impact. There is so much more in life than dieting and I want you to experience it all, unencumbered by the burden of hating your body!

Each of us has our own personal history and influences that led us to this present moment. *The Diet-Free Revolution* starts from where you are, right here, right now, and will help you leave dieting behind once and for all. The weight loss industry convinces us that we need dieting, that we cannot possibly be strong enough to succeed on our own. This is the culture of dependency the industry fosters; although diets don't work, we are deluded into believing that we are doomed without them. We are scolded for "letting" our bodies be imperfect. Our natural differences in shape, size, skin tone, stretch marks, cellulite, and scars become moral failings. *The Diet-Free Revolution* changes this paradigm by encouraging you to accept, love, and care for yourself by replacing messages from the diet industry with messages from the person who knows you the best—you! Trusting yourself is a scary thing to do and requires bravery and perseverance, but the payoff is enormous. And I'll be right here to guide you.

I invite you to throw away your bathroom scale (or at least place it on a very high shelf in a very deep closet in the farthest recesses of your home) for the duration of the program. If you finish this book and remain convinced that dieting or losing weight is the answer, feel free to take down the scale and weigh yourself to your heart's delight. But for this program, you won't need a scale to know what is happening to your body.

Our body comes equipped with sophisticated mechanisms that signal to us when we are hungry, what to eat, and when we've had enough. All of us are wired this way. The problem is that dieting teaches us to ignore our body. Many of us have learned to tune out our inner signals so much that they have become muted. *The Diet-Free Revolution* will help you reconnect with these innate signals by using mindfulness practices to become fully present and aware in your body and with your eating experiences. Instead of attempting to override our body's natural physiology through willpower and dieting, this book helps us work *with* our body's natural physiology without struggle.

The Diet-Free Revolution is divided into ten steps, each designed to help you break free from dieting, reconnect with your body, eat in a peaceful, nurturing way, and start living a life full of satisfaction. Each step builds on the last, gradually creating a solid foundation to change your relationship with food, your body, and yourself. In each chapter you'll find stories, lessons, activities, and meditations to help you fully engage with the program. The ten steps of *The Diet-Free Revolution* are

- Step 1: Say goodbye to dieting

- Step 2: Challenge your assumptions about weight and health

- Step 3: Embrace the power of awareness and learn the five-minute meditation

- Step 4: Treat yourself with compassion and evict your inner critic

- Step 5: Hear and feed your hunger

- Step 6: Find fullness

- Step 7: Embrace your yum by tuning in to taste

- Step 8: Let your body guide you in eating what you want when you want it

- Step 9: Deeply care for your emotional needs

- Step 10: Live a life full of self-care, value, and pleasure

Steps 1 and 2 focus on letting go of dieting. We'll unpack a lot of the research on weight and health and the impact that the diet-industrial complex has on our bodies. If you are eager to jump into the "how-to" part of the program, feel free to skip ahead to step 3, but I encourage you to return to these chapters as they are important. Releasing your attachment to dieting creates space to approach your body differently, with presence and compassion, as you will learn to do in steps 3 and 4. Turning toward your body with awareness and kindness allows you to more clearly hear (and trust) what your body is telling you. You'll need that for steps 5 through 8, which focus on tuning in to the signals your body is sending you to guide your eating—hunger, fullness, taste, urges/cravings, and your body's responses to different foods. Once you are able to honor your body's appetite cues, it becomes easier to identify when you are called to eat for emotional reasons, which we address in step 9. While it is always okay to eat in response to emotions—in fact this can be an important part of healthy eating and also be a pretty darned good coping mechanism during particularly difficult times—it is also important to make sure that you adequately care for your emotional needs. And finally, once you have learned to eat more peacefully in tune with your body, we can shift our focus toward what to do with all that time and energy you've freed up! Step 10 is all about how to embrace the full, pleasurable, values-driven life you deserve.

At the end of each chapter, you will find mindfulness meditations, mindful eating practices, and/or other take-action activities to help you engage more deeply with the material. Some of the take-action activities are journaling prompts; you may choose to use a formal journal for these activities, but any kind of notebook (or even scrap paper!) or the notes application on your phone will serve the purpose. Many of the mindfulness meditations and mindful eating practices can also be found in audio format at www.drconason.com/diet-free-revolution/. While some of the mindful eating practices may be easier to do initially when eating alone, they most certainly can be done while eating with others—often without your dining companions even knowing that you are doing anything different. If it is not your custom to eat alone, or if you simply don't have opportunities for solo meals or snacks, please don't let that deter you from trying the mindful eating practices while dining with others. The intention is for mindful eating to eventually become an integral part of your everyday eating experiences, and for many of us, that includes eating with others.

These strategies are designed to provide a temporary structure, a scaffolding of sorts, to help you transition away from diet culture. When you start this process, it may feel like there is a lot of focus on your eating. You are learning a new skill, so we break it down into the different elements. Imagine taking tennis lessons for the first time. Your instructor teaches you how to grip the racket, position your feet, and watch the ball. It feels incredibly awkward. Paying so much attention to every detail, it's hard to imagine ever being able to hit the ball, let alone play a game. But once you have practiced the drills and gained expertise, it all becomes second nature. You instinctively know how to grasp the racket, your feet place themselves where they need to be on the court, and you become at one with the game. Serena Williams isn't at the US Open thinking about her grip on the racket. Her body knows what to do. Think of the practices in this book as those early tennis lessons. Once you are able to trust your body, listen, and honor what your body is telling you, the structured tools, check-ins, and practices gradually fade away as you start to eat in a way that feels intuitive and instinctual.

In the following chapters, you will meet Tracy, Michael, Mia, and Linda, four people (fictionalized characters, based on composite themes from my clients with a sprinkling of my own personal experiences) from different walks of life brought together in my Anti-Diet Plan group program. Perhaps you will identify with a piece of their story, an aspect of their journey, and feel less alone in your own struggle. And maybe, just maybe, their story will light the path for your own, instilling hope and showing you that, yes, healing and recovery are possible. We are all living in the noxious sludge of diet culture, and that tends to make our struggles more similar than different (although, as mentioned earlier, living in a body marginalized by our culture adds additional layers).

The Diet-Free Revolution will encourage you to eat when you are hungry (and sometimes when you are not), choose foods that you want to eat and make you feel good, and stop when you've had enough. Sound too easy? It's not. This way of eating is alien to most of us. We mistrust our body, our instincts, and ourselves. We criticize our body, ignore our natural signals of hunger, fullness, and satiety, and rely on external sources like diet plans and diet experts to tell us what to eat, when to eat, and how to feel about our bodies. Now we must relearn how to eat attuned with our body. And in order to do that, we must trust our body. *The Diet-Free Revolution* will show you the way.

A Note on Language and Identity

Throughout this book, I use the term *fat*. In alliance with the fat acceptance movement, I use *fat* as a neutral descriptor of body size. There is a movement to reclaim the word *fat* and remove the negative associations from it. It is in this spirit that I use this word.

I recognize that, for many people, this term is anything but neutral. The word *fat* is often associated with memories of trauma, abuse, bullying, pain, and harm. I want to honor that experience as well. In my work with clients, I use the words they choose to describe their bodies. In a book, that is obviously not possible. The language that I use to describe certain bodies may not be the language that you use to describe your own body. I support each individual in choosing how to describe and identify their own body. For this book, I made the choice to use language consistent with the fat acceptance movement, as it centers the voices of people who have experienced oppression based on body size and represents the language this group uses. In addition to *fat*, I also use the terms *higher-weight*, *larger-bodied*, and *living in a larger body*. Although these terms are also not perfect—and center a standard weight or size that these bodies are above and/or connote a separation from one's body, as if it were a house that can be moved into or out of—I use them because they are also commonly used within the fat acceptance community.

Wherever possible, I avoid using the terms *overweight* and *obese*. While some people may think these terms are more socially acceptable than *fat*, they are inherently stigmatizing. *Overweight* means that there is one ideal range of weight and you are over it. In contrast, *The Diet-Free Revolution* espouses that bodies are meant to exist at a diverse range of shapes and sizes, and one is not more inherently valuable than the other. *Obese* is a medical term that pathologizes fat bodies as sick bodies. This idea is also counter to the philosophy of *The Diet-Free Revolution*, which affirms that health is possible across the weight spectrum. On occasion, when discussing research studies or quoting other people, you may see the terms *overweight* and *obesity* used to maintain the integrity of the primary sources.

I am a white thin-privileged heterosexual cisgender (meaning the sex assigned to me at birth is consistent with my gender identity) woman. I live in an able body and don't use any accommodations to navigate the world around me. My parents were both college educated, and I've had class and financial privileges throughout my life. These multiple privileges don't mean that I haven't had hardships or difficult experiences—like all of us, I have. And this doesn't mean that if you are a thin-privileged white woman, your life hasn't been hard. It doesn't mean that you haven't struggled with body image or an eating disorder or hating yourself or trauma or being bullied for your body or any of the other challenges that come up on the road of life. It just means that you haven't experienced systemic oppression due to your race or body size. While life hasn't always been easy, I haven't had hardships because of my race, body size, sexual orientation, gender identity, disability, or educational, financial, and class statuses. I don't know firsthand what it is like to navigate the world as a fat person or a Black person or a queer person or as anything other than a thin-privileged white woman. In my therapy practice, I work primarily with other white women—many of whom are larger-bodied—who are, for the most part, also cisgender and straight. I have been honored to be able to hear their stories and know their lives. Through my work as a therapist, I have gained a glimpse into what life is like for some people in larger bodies. But this by no means gives me a first-person understanding of what life is like for fat people. I can only write from my own position in the world, and that inevitably means that my writing is limited. The best that I can do is acknowledge that and hope you will find some usefulness from my perspective on these issues.

A Disclaimer

This book is not intended to be a replacement for medical or psychiatric treatment. If you are struggling with an eating disorder, I highly recommend working with a treatment team to assess whether this book is appropriate for your treatment. Some of the content in this book could be triggering, including stories of people struggling with eating disorders and disordered eating and mentions of calories and weight when discussing research studies. If you are struggling with an eating disorder and in need of a treatment team, you can find a list of providers who identify as weight-inclusive on my website at www.drconason.com/diet-free-revolution/ or by calling the National Eating Disorders Association at (800) 931-2237 or visiting their website (www.nationaleatingdisorders.org). If you feel triggered or dysregulated by any of the content in this book, I recommend consulting with a licensed mental health professional.

1

STEP 1: Say Goodbye to Dieting (and Hello to Happiness!)

inda, a sixty-nine-year-old high-powered music executive, entered my office with an energy that demanded attention. Her short hair was dyed fiery red, and she wore thick oversized glasses that glittered with little rhinestones at the corners. She was dressed all in black, layers of structured material draping over her body. The billowy fabric made it hard to tell where Linda started and the garments ended.

"I have so much weight to lose," she lamented at our first meeting. "I don't know what's wrong with me. I've tried every diet plan out there, but I just can't seem to get this weight off." Her voice was filled with anger, but her eyes betrayed her as they welled up with tears that she quickly blinked away.

Linda held out her phone to show me a picture. "Look at what I used to be!" I glanced down at the image on the screen and thought for a moment it was vintage Cher before realizing it was a picture of Linda. Her hair is jet black and winds down past her slim waist, which is exposed in a suede fringed crop top with matching low-rise pants. She is standing with the Rolling Stones. "This was at Andy Warhol's Christmas party in 1973. I was really something, right? Look how thin and beautiful I was. And look at what's happened." She gestured toward her perfectly lovely body. "I'm old and fat. I used to be a mover and shaker. Now everything on my body is moving and shaking in the wrong places." She chuckled, which did little to hide her deep sadness. "My office is filled with pretty young things nipping at my heels, waiting for me to drop dead or retire so they can snag my corner office. My new boss is trying to push me out. He's half my age and is always talking about staying fresh. He probably thinks I'm about as fresh as spoiled milk." She giggled again, in a way that felt mechanical and mis-matched to the troubling situation she was describing. "They don't want old hags like me talking to new talent. Sex sells and I'm fifty years over sexy. They want a hot twenty-something who the clients want to be seen on the town with, who will work twice as hard for half the pay, and who knows the latest social media trends. I'm still trying to figure out Facebook." She laughed again. I got the visual image of Linda ice skating, her humor serv-ing as a thin layer of ice she glides over, trying desperately to avoid any cracks lest she fall into an abyss of pain. "These kids, they will work all day and night. I just don't have the stamina for that anymore. Especially with this extra weight I'm carrying. I'm so tired."

Linda went on to describe the anti-inflammatory diet that her doctor promised would help her arthritis and keep away the cancer she had been diagnosed with seven years before. She was convinced that if she could sub-sist on a diet of vegetables and lean protein, she would stave off this horrid aging process. But adhering to this strict diet proved impossible, which was why she came to my office. Instead of vegetables and lean protein, Linda found herself gorging on donuts and cream puffs. "I have no self-control. Why can't I just get it together? It's sickening!"

Linda started in the music industry as an intern when she was nineteen years old. From there, she worked her way through the ranks to her current position as one of the top executives at her label. This was a feat for anyone, but especially for a woman in this male-dominated field. As one of the hardest working employees in the company, she knew no one could accuse her of being unmotivated or lazy.

Linda's life sounded glamorous. She attended parties with celebrities, hung out backstage at concerts, and got invited to all the most exclusive events. Her stories drew me in with salacious details about Hollywood star-lets and rock stars, but I tried to stay focused on why Linda was coming to see me: to resolve these awful feelings she had about her body. Linda was plagued by a harsh inner bully who tagged along as her plus-one. *Look at that woman—she is so much younger and thinner than you. And she is only eating a salad instead of shoving food in her face like you do. You wonder why you're fat? It's because you obviously have no discipline!* Her inner critic was relentless.

Eating was the one area of Linda's life where she did not feel successful or satisfied. She described a happy marriage, a good relationship with her adult daughter, and fulfilling friendships. While her job was exhausting, she took pride in her success and enjoyed her career. She just could not seem to get a handle on her weight. Linda had started noticing the pounds creep on as she aged and, for the past thirty years, tried unsuccessfully to lose weight.

Linda had tried just about every diet plan imaginable—and even some that I couldn't imagine! Eat no carbs. Eat only bran muffins. Eat no red meat. Eat only steak. Eat no sugar. Eat only chocolate. Linda had tried diets named after foods: The Grapefruit Diet, The Cabbage Soup Diet, The Vinegar Diet, and The Cookie Diet. She tried diets named after luxurious places: The South Beach Diet, The Scarsdale Diet, The Hamptons Diet, and The Mediterranean Diet. She had tried diets named after famous doc-tors: The Atkins Diet, The Dukan Diet, The Stillman Diet, and The Ornish Diet. She had cleansed, detoxified, acupunctured, and hypnotized herself in pursuit of weight loss. But no matter what she did, she just couldn't seem to win the battle against her own body.

"It works for a few weeks and then I fall off the wagon. I just can't stick to it. I don't understand, I put my all into everything I do—my work, marriage, friendships—but I can't seem to pull it together around food."

I asked Linda to tell me more about her struggles. She sagged into her chair as though the mere thought of it weighed a ton. "I try to follow the anti-inflammatory diet my doctor recommended; that means no carbs, no sugar, no red meat, and no processed foods. But sweets are my downfall!

I love dessert, but I really try to avoid it. Sugar is a big no-no. The problem is, I'm a chocoholic."

Linda tried to cope with her food issues by limiting the foods she kept in her home. No breads, pastas, sweets, packaged foods, or meat would cross over the threshold to her apartment. While this plan seldom works for anyone, it was especially ineffective for Linda because her job forced her to dine out several times a week. She wined and dined at the top restaurants in Manhattan. Linda viewed dining out as a special occasion, even though she ate out more often than she ate in. And special occasions meant that she got to cheat on her diet. So Linda gorged on the finest breads, pastas, and desserts Manhattan chefs had to offer. How could she resist?

Heaps of remorse followed these dinners. She would leave the meal feeling uncomfortably stuffed and bloated, with her inner mean girl taunting her all the way home. *How could you eat all of that? You are such a pig!* Linda went to bed full of delicious sweets and regret. To console herself, she would vow to be better tomorrow. *I won't eat any carbs at all. Only fat-free yogurt, fruits, and vegetables. Maybe I should do a juice cleanse? That will help me get back on track.* She felt empowered with these thoughts, excited at the prospect of regaining control over her eating. But it never lasted for long.

I asked, "Is it possible that dieting is the *problem* rather than the solution?" Linda looked at me as if I had just suggested that the sky may actually be red instead of blue. As a therapist, I have perfected the poker face. I raised my eyebrows to convey that I would not be easily deterred and waited for her answer. Her eyes narrowed as she started to really think about the question. "Well, I guess anything is possible," she said hesitantly after a few minutes of silence. Dieting had so obviously been the answer that she had never questioned it before. Together we started to explore her history with dieting. While she had lost weight in the past, she would always regain the weight—plus extra pounds—within months of ending the diet. For this she blamed herself. "I get lazy," she said when asked about this weight loss–weight gain cycle. "I'm able to stay disciplined for a few weeks, even sometimes a few months, but then I give into my gluttonous desires. I just need to figure out a way to stay motivated." After everything that Linda had shared about her life, it was hard for me to believe that she was a woman who lacked motivation or discipline.

I posed a thought-provoking question: "Is it possible that diets inherently involve both sides of the weight loss–weight gain coin? Could the weight regain be a natural part of the diet cycle?" We looked at research studies (which I'll summarize for you in the next section) documenting the failures of dieting and the tendency for diets to lead to long-term weight gain. We talked about the financial incentives that the weight loss industry has in selling us the message that we need to diet and the cultural pressures for women to stay preoccupied with changing their bodies. We discussed ageism in our culture and the impossible demands on women to be young, thin, and beautiful to be relevant, powerful, and valued. We explored Linda's fears around aging, death, and her changing identity. And we raised the possibility that her body was not inherently flawed. As we had these conversations over the first few months of therapy, I could practically see Linda's brain cranking away, struggling to see a familiar pattern in a new light.

As Linda began to accept that dieting was the problem rather than the solution, she initially felt despondent and panicked, "If dieting won't help me, then what will?"

"Don't worry," I assured her. "There is another way."

Linda joined my group program, where she met weekly with me and the other participants to work her way through the steps that you will learn in this book. As she heard the stories of the other participants and how they too struggled to stick to a diet, it really clicked for her. The whole paradigm was rigged. The diet industry, bolstered by patriarchal messaging, had convinced Linda that her appetite was leading her astray in her quest for weight loss and health. Every time she fell prey to a warm doughy dinner roll, perfectly al dente penne, or decadent chocolate lava cake, she saw the problem as her body, her weak will, or her lack of motivation. Dieting fueled her inner critic, who would berate her endlessly, convincing her that her only hope for salvation was to return to dieting. What a cruel farce!

In our weekly group meetings, Linda and the other members questioned the efficacy of diets and examined the good, bad, and ugly of their past experiences. We did exercises, similar to the ones you'll find at the end of each chapter in this book, to increase Linda's awareness of her harsh inner voice and learn how to talk back to—and eventually quiet—this voice. As she hushed this critical voice, another one began to emerge in Linda's head—a compassionate voice that supported her in caring for her body with kindness. Over time she was able to see that her *diet* was leading her astray, *not her own body*.

It was hard for Linda to let go of the idea that her life would be better if she could lose weight. "But surely my knees wouldn't ache so bad if I didn't have all this extra weight on me! Plus I can't even buy clothes in a regular store anymore. I can only get my size online and, ugh, it just kills me to buy clothes in such an enormous size. I feel so old and frumpy all the time." It was hard for me to argue with Linda about this. Would her life be easier if she lost weight? Probably. It's a lot easier to live in a smaller body in our fatphobic culture. But, as you will learn in this chapter and the next, the problem is not Linda's body (just as the problem is not your body). The problem is our culture. Besides, it was becoming abundantly clear to Linda, from both the research we were learning about and her own lived experiences, that we really don't have an effective way for people to lose weight and keep it off long-term.

"Why do you want to lose weight?" I asked Linda.

"I want to be able to move without pain," she said immediately. "I want to be able to go into a store and know that they'll have my size. I don't want to have to hide my body all the time. I want men to look at me again. I want to be young," she said, with a laugh. I reflected on how Linda had become less reliant on the humor that was omnipresent at the start of our work together, although it still made an appearance every now and again.

"I unfortunately haven't mastered the art of aging reversal yet, although I hear there is a wizardry office around the corner that will take a lot of your money for that service," I said jokingly, thinking of the plastic surgery center on my block with a prominent sign claiming to reverse aging.

"Let's look at what you really want." After some more discussion, Linda was able to identify improved mobility, less pain, and feeling better about her body as her underlying goals. We explored how she could work toward her goals now in her current body. She began physical therapy to treat her knee pain, as well as acupuncture as recommended by her doctor, and she invested in new clothes that she felt more stylish in. She grieved the loss of the fantasized body that she longed for, and worked on accepting her body exactly as it was at that very moment, even if she didn't always like it (you'll learn more about body acceptance in chapter 4). Through this work, Linda shifted her goals away from weight loss to focus on the things that she really wanted in life. This allowed her to get her life off pause and stop waiting for that magical day when she would reach her goal weight to feel better about her body and her health. She felt empowered as she started to focus on behaviors that were more in her control, versus changing her body size, which was out of her control.

Breaking up with diets allowed Linda to find a new path toward health, peace, and well-being. Are *you* ready to end your dysfunctional relationship with dieting?

Why Diets Don't Work

Accepting that diets don't work is the first step toward healing our relationship with food. It allows us to embark on this program with an open mind. We must accept that dieting is the *problem* rather than the solution to our struggles. Dieting keeps us stuck in the delusions that our bodies are flawed and that we are helpless to care for ourselves. It binds us in cycles of disordered eating and fuels our inner critic. As long as we believe the false assumption that dieting is the path to salvation, we remain caught in a toxic relationship with dieting that encourages disordered eating, poor health, and shame.

What Is a Diet?

In my office I often meet with clients who tell me that they aren't dieting. Debbie, who recently came to see me for a consultation session, is a typical example. "I'm not on a diet. I just try to eat healthy," she stated firmly. I asked her what "eating healthy" meant, and she rattled off a long list of foods and macronutrients that are restricted. "I try not to eat processed foods …" she started off. "Carbs are inflammatory so I try and avoid those, along with sugar because it's also inflammatory plus it's addictive and once I start with sugar I'm totally out of control, fruit is basically just candy so I try and stay clear except I do allow myself some blueberries on occasion, nightshades are toxic so no eggplant for me even though it used to be my favorite, I don't eat any red meat, I try to eat organic as much as possible …" Debbie went on for several more minutes listing all the foods on the naughty list as she described her not-a-diet diet. Dieting has become so normalized as a way of life that many of us are dieting and don't even think we are dieting.

In recent years, dieting has fallen out of vogue. As the general public became increasingly savvy to the fact that diets don't work, the diet industry scrambled to rebrand itself, hiding under the guise of "wellness" and "health." "It's not a diet, it's a lifestyle change! It's just healthy eating!" diet companies proclaim, trying to convince us that they are all about health, not weight loss, despite promising customers that they will lose weight. These companies are smart and spend tons of money on market research; they know, despite all of our disillusionment with dieting, people still want to lose weight, and if they convince us we can do that without "dieting" customers will flock back. SlimFast and Atkins have given way to cold-pressed juices, raw food meal delivery services, boutique fitness classes, detoxes, "clean eating," even jade eggs for people's vaginas! The wellness industry is largely unregulated; many products don't live up to the hype, and some can be downright dangerous—or a scam. Don't get me wrong, the same old diet companies are still there; it just may be harder to recognize them.

Weight Watchers is one of the most public examples of the rebrand from dieting to wellness. In 2018, after fifty-six years, the company changed its name from "Weight Watchers" to "WW," adopted a new tagline ("wellness that works"), and tried to gaslight us all into believing that they were no longer a diet company—now they're a wellness company. Noom, a diet company whose program regularly recommends people eat fewer calories than the daily recommended intake for a toddler, bills itself as an "anti-diet." We are told that "strong is the new skinny" and "healthy is the new skinny," but when we look at the images of wellness culture (read: young, thin, white, conventionally attractive cis women), one thing is really clear: skinny is the new skinny. *Health* has just become a code word for *thin*.

This new brand of "wellness" is out of reach for most of us. Who can regularly afford boutique fitness classes at $45 a pop or $15 kale chia smoothies or a $66 jade egg for their vagina? It becomes an aspirational ideal that only the most privileged among us have any chance of approximating. Access to "health" (and the veneration that comes from pursuing health) varies across the socioeconomic spectrum, with health and class inextricably linked. Income is one of the largest determinants of health.[1] There is also a strong association between income and body size in the US, with lower socioeconomic status associated with higher body mass index (BMI), especially for women.[2] The moralization of health—and the idea that people in larger bodies are somehow not deserving of respect because they are "unhealthy"—is a comment not just on fatness, but also on class and race. I'll be talking more about health, body size, and the intersections with class, income, and race in chapter 2.

For the purposes of this book, I define a diet as any means of restricting your food intake based on a set of outside rules for the purposes of weight loss, "wellness," or "health." While certain medical conditions may require you to eat in different ways, it is possible to accommodate these needs without overriding your body's inner signals (as I discuss in chapter 8 in the section "Mindful Eating and Chronic Health Conditions"). Dieting means we prioritize messages from the weight loss industry while ignoring messages from our own body. Dieting refers not only to the following of a specific commercial plan but also to a broader "diet mentality" that tells us that certain foods are good or bad and that we are good or bad based on the foods we consume. Our self-worth becomes determined by what we eat; our moral value rises with lettuce and falls with pizza. Who we are and what we do is eclipsed by what we eat and what our bodies look like.

If you have a list of foods that are good/bad, clean/toxic, restricted/permitted, if you judge yourself as being good or bad based on what you eat, if you try to avoid entire food groups, if you feel guilty after eating, or if you decide what to eat or not eat based on an external set of rules, you are most likely on a diet. Most of us are on some kind of a diet. To be raised in diet culture and *not* have a dysfunctional relationship with food is a rare experience.

Not dieting doesn't mean that we must eat all foods or that we don't have certain ways of eating that feel best in our body. It just means that we are eating in accordance with our body and letting our internal signals be our guide. This way of eating tends to be flexible, peaceful, and compassionate. In chapter 8 we'll learn all about how to make choices around food in a way that feels good to our body. Being anti-diet does not mean that we are anti-health. Although health is not a moral imperative (despite what our culture would have us believe) and we are all deserving of respect regardless of health status, if you want to improve your health, there are plenty of ways to do that without dieting.

As we move away from dieting, we will notice how incessant diet mentality is. It's hard to unlearn all the food rules we have internalized. These rules can become deeply ingrained in our brain—I find those Weight Watchers points to be particularly insidious! In chapter 3 we will learn how to practice mindfulness, a technique that can help us be more aware of when these rules arise, so we can observe and recognize them, not as truths to live by but as remnants of diet culture that are not serving us in a healthy way.

Research on Dieting

Most of us are already familiar with the idea that diets don't work. Just think back on your past experiences. Have diets worked for you long-term? If you are reading this book, I'm going to hazard a guess that diets have not solved your problems once and for all. For the vast majority of people, they won't. In 1959 a research study was published that suggested 95 percent of diets fail.[3] More recent research indicates that between 80 and 94 percent of dieters fail to achieve long-term weight loss and maintenance.[4] In fact, the most predictable long-term outcome of dieting may be weight *gain*.[5]

Even the research touted by the weight loss industry as evidence of dieting success paints a pretty bleak picture. The Look AHEAD (Action for Health in Diabetes) trial is often cited as a landmark study that people *can* lose and maintain weight long-term.[6] Its researchers asked participants to diet and exercise and provided them with a ton of support—stuff the average dieter doesn't have access to, like group and individual counseling sessions, monitoring and support from the research staff, provision of meal replacements, detailed customized meal plans and menus, access to exercise classes and support in developing an exercise routine, and, in some cases, even the purchasing of gym memberships, home exercise equipment, personal training sessions, and weight loss medications.[7] When participants inevitably regained weight during the study's nine-year observation period, they received even more support and were given access to more interventions like weight loss medications, more intensive counseling, and new behavior-change strategies. Even with all of that, participants still didn't clear the researchers' own benchmark for weight loss success. After approximately nine years in the study, participants maintained a mere 5 percent weight loss, falling short of the researchers' stated goal of 7 percent weight loss.[8]

That's a lot of work that people went through—focusing on restricting their eating every single day, ongoing counseling to maintain the diet, meal replacement shakes, diet pills, exercising, tracking, and weighing—all to maintain a weight loss far less than most dieters hope for. The fact that this study is one of the best available to provide evidence that people can maintain weight loss long-term speaks to how elusive long-term weight loss really is. These are the best possible results with the most resources available. I wonder what happened to the participants after the study ended and they no longer had access to all those resources?

Dieting success stories are so uncommon that researchers created an online database to study the rare unicorns who have been able to lose and maintain weight loss long-term. The National Weight Control

Registry (NWCR) includes over 10,000 "success" stories of people (including people who have undergone weight loss surgery) who have managed to lose at least thirty pounds and keep the weight off for at least one year.[9] Fat activist Ragen Chastain explains in her blog *Dances with Fat* that when we consider how many people in the US diet each year (which she estimates at 45–80 million people, likely a low estimate), the NWCR represents less than 1 percent of all dieters.[10] Yet the other 99 percent of dieters think this 1 percent is the norm and are convinced it is their own fault they keep failing their diets. Does anyone else see fault in this logic?

What's more, when we look closely at the rare "success stories" on the NWCR, we start to see that maybe the behaviors they are engaging in aren't so healthy after all. People on the registry spend hours at the gym, track every calorie, and think about food and their body nonstop. They follow an incredibly rigid restricted diet, and they experience weight gain if they even slightly deviate from their diet. A 2017 study observed that people on the NWCR are engaging in the same types of behaviors observed in patients diagnosed with chronic anorexia nervosa.[11] The authors of that study stopped short of suggesting that the people on the NWCR have an eating disorder and instead suggest that we may be able to apply the symptoms observed in thin people with chronic anorexia to unlock the secrets of long-term weight loss in fat people. As psychologist Deb Burgard observes, "We prescribe for fat people what we diagnose as eating disordered in thin people" (personal communication, October 13, 2020).

Why *don't* diets work? It turns out that there are a lot of psychological and biological factors that make falling off the wagon and regaining weight pretty much inevitable. Let's look at the research, starting with some of the early studies.

In 1944 physiologist Ancel Keys studied thirty-six mentally and physically healthy young men to examine the effects of calorie restriction in what came to be known as the Minnesota Starvation Study.[12] They were supposed to lose 25 percent of their body weight and went through different phases of calorie restriction. In the most restrictive phase, participants were fed just over 1,500 calories daily, a similar allotment to many of today's popular diet plans. What the men experienced may not come as a surprise to anyone who has been on a diet: They became obsessed with food. They dreamed about food, talked about food, collected recipes, and compulsively read cookbooks. In addition to thinking about food all the time, participants reported fatigue, weakness, loss of sex drive, irritability, and depression. When the men in the study were given more access to food in the rehabilitation phase, many started binge eating (defined today as eating an unusually large amount of food in a discrete period of time, typically less than two hours, accompanied by a sense of loss of control).[13] Remember, these were all healthy men with no prior history of food issues or an eating disorder. This study is a clear example of how restricting our food intake—as we do when we are dieting—makes us more preoccupied with food and more prone to binge eating. Rather than a lack of willpower, this is our body's healthy response to keep us fed, nourished, and alive.

In 1975 researchers C. Peter Herman and Deborah Mack developed "restraint theory" to explain why diets fail.[14] Based on a series of experiments, restraint theory posits that because dieters rely on cognitive control (what we commonly think of as willpower or self-discipline) rather than physiological cues to govern eating behavior, they must create rules to control their intake. These rules usually include specifications of permissible and forbidden foods. Dieters are vulnerable to overeating when cognitive controls are disrupted by emotions, consumption of a forbidden food, or perception of having overeaten. When dieters eat a forbidden food, they experience what the researchers called the "what the hell" effect. As in, *what the hell, I've already blown my diet by eating one slice of pizza* (or any other forbidden food), *I might as well eat the whole pie.*

Paradoxically, attempting to restrict food intake through dieting *induces* excessive eating and loss of control over food intake.[15] As most dieters know, cognitive control isn't a very effective strategy for governing our eating. And why would it be? Cognitive control was never intended to rule over our appetite. As you'll learn in this book, your body already has a very efficient appetite regulation system uniquely designed to guide your eating that doesn't require any willpower or discipline.

Dieting encourages "all or none" thinking (i.e., the "what the hell" effect), feelings of deprivation, guilt, shame, and mistrust in our bodies. We hear our stomach growling and think, *I shouldn't be hungry now; I already ate lunch.* If we have a craving for chocolate, we deny ourselves what we crave because it is "unhealthy" or not on our diet plan. Alternatively we decide that we'll be "bad" today and break our diet by eating chocolate cake. We eat a lot of the cake, regardless of whether we want it, because what we don't eat today will be restricted tomorrow. This "last meal mentality" is common in dieting—it feels like we have to eat all we can now, while it's available to us, before it becomes off-limits again. After all, we already blew our diet, why stop now? Caught in so much conflict, we often don't notice the taste of the food or what we really want, and it is hard to stop eating when we've had enough. Only when we ditch the destructive dieting mentality can we truly eat in harmony with our body. We'll learn more about nonrestrictive eating and how it allows us to overcome last meal mentality in chapter 8.

Research Confirms: Our Body Is Amazing

Much to the chagrin of dieters seeking to lose weight, our body is designed to keep our weight stable, especially to ensure that our weight doesn't get too low. When we lose weight, a complex series of events is set into action to encourage us to regain the weight. This strong biological system was developed over eons of evolution to keep us alive during times of famine. That's a good thing. We want to stay alive, and our body needs to be nourished to run well. As we'll see soon when we dig into the research on "set point theory," fighting against our own body is a losing battle. Our cognitive control system, which dieting relies on, is no match for our biology. That's why psychological techniques for behavior change do not help people lose weight—our body size is not a behavior. As much as we are taught to exert control over our body, our body is actually meant to guide *us* (not the other way around). When we can stop interfering in what our body is naturally meant to do, we have a much easier time of things.

Our weight is regulated by an intricate system of processes that operates like a thermostat. When you set the thermostat in your home or car to your desired temperature, let's say 69 degrees, it will work to maintain that temperature, turning on and off the heater or air conditioner if the temperature goes above or below 69 degrees. Our body operates similarly. When our weight drops below what's comfortable for our body (our "set point" weight range), the thermostat turns on, activating an intertwined system of hormones that controls our appetite and metabolism.

Metabolism is the rate at which our body breaks down the food we eat and turns it into energy for important life-sustaining functions like breathing, thinking, and moving (isn't our body amazing!?). When we restrict our food intake, as we do when dieting, our metabolism slows down, requiring fewer calories for our body to run. The human body is great at adapting; when we aren't adequately nourishing our body, it finds a way to make do with less, even if that means functioning suboptimally. This is why we may notice that we have less energy, feel more irritable, and can't think as clearly when we are on a diet (remember the men from the Ancel Keys starvation study?).

In 1995 Rudolph Leibel and his colleagues at Rockefeller University published a groundbreaking study about set point theory in the *New England Journal of Medicine* that changed the way we understand what happens in our bodies when we diet and lose weight.[16] The study included eighteen "obese" and twenty-three "never-obese" participants who were admitted to the inpatient unit of the hospital and studied extensively in a controlled environment. Participants were kept secluded in the hospital for anywhere between three months and two years.[17] The lean participants, mostly students who also worked at the hospital's research lab, were paid $40 per day for participating and tended to check out of the study after a few months. On the other hand, the "obese" participants were paid only with the hope of weight loss, and many stayed confined in the hospital for years working toward this goal. Participants in the study were given a liquid diet and "underfed" to lose 10 to 20 percent of their body weight. I can't help but imagine the desperation of someone who would agree to give up everything in their life to live in a hospital for two years in exchange for the promise of weight loss. Living in a fat body in our fatphobic world is brutal.

Results of this study indicated that people who had reduced their weight through dieting, so it fell below their set point range, required far fewer calories (about 250–400 calories less) to maintain their body weight than would be expected for someone of the same body size who hadn't reduced their weight. In other words, metabolism slows after weight loss, so the body becomes more efficient at holding on to energy and thus requires fewer calories to maintain a lower body weight. Besides these metabolic adaptations, this research also revealed that for people who have dropped below their set point weight range, their body sends other signals to make them feel hungrier, have more intense food cravings, and regain weight. Participants also reported physical discomfort at the reduced body weight, including a feeling of dysphoria, that was alleviated by weight regain. Our weight-regulation system seems to operate like an on-off switch that is not necessarily proportional to the amount of weight lost. Once a certain amount of weight is lost and we cross the lower threshold of our set point range, our body's thermostat kicks into gear.

A 2016 study of contestants from the television show *The Biggest Loser* built on this earlier research about set point theory.[18] For those of you fortunate enough to be unfamiliar with the show, *The Biggest Loser* is a reality show in which fat people are subjected to torturous exercise routines while being berated by a personal trainer, put on low-calorie diets, and asked to share their deepest personal traumas on national television. This study wasn't the first to research this program; a 2012 study showed that the mere viewing of *The Biggest Loser* was associated with increased anti-fat attitudes in viewers.[19] In the 2016 study, researchers from the National Institutes of Health (NIH) assessed contestants six years after the show was filmed and found that participants had significantly slower resting metabolism than when the show started. This shouldn't come as a surprise, since we already know that dieting and weight loss slow down our metabolism. But this study showed that six years after their initial weight loss, the participants' metabolisms still hadn't returned to what they were before the show. Despite having regained significant weight—some contestants were even at a higher weight than before the show—their metabolisms had not recovered.

Similar to Leibel's 1995 study, the 2016 *Biggest Loser* study found that not only did participants require far fewer calories to maintain their current weight, but also their body was sending them signals to increase their appetite. Leptin, sometimes referred to as the "satiety hormone," is released by our fat cells based on how much we've eaten and signals our brain that we've had enough to eat. It's like the off switch for hunger. At the season finale of *The Biggest Loser,* when contestants were at their lowest weights, their levels of leptin (which were normal prior to starting the show) were almost zero. Without leptin, they would never feel satisfied and always want to keep eating more. Leptin levels increased over time as contestants regained weight, but at the six-year follow-up point, they still weren't back up to where they were before the show. Prior research studies also reported people had lower leptin levels following weight loss, along with other hormonal changes including increased levels of ghrelin.[20] The "hunger hormone" produced in your gut, ghrelin signals your brain that it's time to eat. Increased ghrelin levels after weight loss mean that people who are at a reduced body weight feel much hungrier than people who are at their set point weight.

In addition to metabolic and hormonal changes, increased cravings are also experienced by dieters. Research suggests that depriving yourself of certain foods increases your cravings for those very same foods. The cravings reported by dieters are more frequent, more intense, more difficult to resist, and slower to disappear than cravings experienced by non-dieters. One study found that dieters eventually eat the restricted foods in about 70 percent of the instances that they experience a craving.[21] Interestingly, when dieters finally cave and eat the craved foods, they don't experience increased enjoyment of the food. So if you are on a diet, you may not even take pleasure in that tempting slice of chocolate cake you had been dreaming about all day. This lack of enjoyment likely stems from the emotional conflicts around food that make it difficult to be present and relish the taste. Guilt really can spoil a meal.

To summarize, dieting relies on our cognitive control system. This is what we commonly think of as motivation, willpower, and discipline—all the reasons we blame ourselves when we go off-track with our diet. This cognitive system was never designed to govern our eating, and it is simply no match for the powerful biological appetite and weight-regulation systems designed to keep us alive. When we diet and lose weight, our body lowers our metabolism, reducing the number of calories needed to maintain (and subsequently gain) weight. Our body also sends out signals that make us feel hungrier and less satisfied, and they trigger intense cravings for food. These factors combine to make it nearly impossible in the long term to maintain weight loss through dieting. Do you still think it's your fault that you can't stick to your diet?

If you are still committed to the idea that losing weight is the only path to health and happiness, this may all sound pessimistic. But stay with me here. I'm not telling you all of this to be a Debbie Downer. Quite the contrary, I'm sharing this information so that you can stop engaging in a paradigm that does not work. It is much easier to extricate yourself from dieting when you realize that it doesn't even work. Not a little bit. The system is inherently flawed. It's all a sham.

As Rudolph Leibel, the prominent "obesity" researcher and author of the 1995 set point study, said in an interview with Charlie Rose, "[Weight regain] is not a question of willpower per se, it's a question of metabolism. The metabolism has adjusted in such a way to make it virtually inevitable … that the individual will regain the weight … Biology is the major dictate of body composition … [weight] is biology the way that height, skin color, eye color, hair color are, and should be treated that way."[22] You don't need to continue the endless battle against your own biology. You haven't failed. Your body is not bad. In fact, your body is simply doing exactly what it was built to do.

If you are worried that you have permanently "messed up" your body through dieting, remember that our bodies are nothing if not adaptable and resilient. If you have a chronic history of dieting and weight cycling (losing and regaining weight again and again), it may take a little longer to connect with your innate signals of hunger and fullness. But I assure you they are there. While most of my clients worry that their body doesn't have these signals or is "too broken" to eat mindfully, this rarely pans out to be true. In almost all instances, using the tools outlined in this book, people have been able to reconnect with their body to hear their internal signals to guide their eating. That's not to say that you may not need extra support in the form of psychotherapy or nutritional counseling, depending on the severity of what has been going on with your body (and almost always in the case of someone struggling with an eating disorder). For that reason, I provide a list of providers who practice from a philosophy aligned with *The Diet-Free Revolution* on my website (www.drconason.com /diet-free-revolution/).

The dance that our body does to help us regulate our body weight is an important function of health. Protecting our set point weight is just one of the countless incredible things that our body does to keep us alive. Our body is wise. It may not always do what we want it to do, but it is doing what it needs to do. If you are unhappy with your body size, that makes sense. We live in a culture with pervasive fatphobia and weight-based discrimination. In the next chapter we are going to explore the origins of these ideas that fatness is bad, unhealthy, and undesirable. It is hard to live in our world in a larger body. Always remember, the problem is diet culture, not your body.

TAKE-ACTION ACTIVITIES

Journal about your relationship with dieting

Answer the following questions:

- In what ways have diets worked for you, and in what ways have diets failed you?

- Are you ready to say goodbye to dieting? Be honest with yourself. It's okay if you aren't ready yet. In fact, it's important to acknowledge that. Dieting offers tastes of the good along with the bad, which can make it hard to part ways. There is a lot invested in convincing us that we need dieting.

- If you aren't ready to say goodbye, are you ready to take a break from dieting for the duration of this program?

Write a breakup letter to dieting

(Or a "we are taking a break" letter if you aren't ready to say goodbye for good.) Try to identify both the positive and negative aspects of dieting. How has dieting helped you, and how has dieting hurt you? Think about the good times and the bad. Be sure to consider the full diet cycle, both when you are on the plan and when you go off. Are the lists lopsided? What feelings come up when you think about not dieting? What are the fantasies or hopes that you are holding onto about dieting? This letter should end with a final goodbye or a "let's take a break," whichever you feel more comfortable with.

One of the key elements of this exercise is to identify both your positive and negative associations to dieting. We wouldn't diet if it wasn't serving us in some way, and we wouldn't be reading this book if it wasn't harming us in some way. It is important to identify both sides of the conflict so that we can process our complicated feelings about dieting and move on with our life!

List your fears about not dieting

Write down what you worry will happen if you don't diet—"I'll be completely out of control, I'll gain a ton of weight, I'll binge nonstop, I'll feel lost," or whatever you're feeling. Now go through this list again and make a check mark next to each item that also occurs *with* the dieting cycle—feeling out of control? Check! Weight loss followed by weight gain? Check!

List your reasons for wanting to lose weight

If you have the goal of losing weight, write down why you want to lose weight. Then go back over this list and mark each item that can be met independent of weight loss. For example, you may have listed "have more self-confidence" as a motivation. Is it possible to increase self-confidence in any way other than weight loss? Hint: quieting your harsh inner critic and being more compassionate toward yourself usually helps. If you listed "improve my health," consider: are there any ways that I can work toward improving my health now, in my current body? In chapter 2 we'll use this list again and learn all about ways to improve health that don't involve losing weight.

The "thin picture" exercise

Have you ever weighed less than you currently do? If so, find a picture of you at your lower weight. This could be either a photograph or a mental image. Journal about what your life was like at that time. Try to remember this period as fully as possible and imagine yourself back there. What were you doing to achieve this lower weight? Were you truly happy? Did you feel emotionally fulfilled? Were you living a life of pleasure, enjoyment, and satisfaction? Or did you still not feel good about your body? Did you still want to lose a few more pounds? Did you socially isolate yourself? Were you preoccupied with food, dieting, and exercise? Was the regimen or weight loss sustainable? And if so, was there an associated cost? What was the process by which you regained the weight? You may also want to take some time to mourn the loss of that thinner body and the privileges you may have been granted as a result. Try to allow yourself to feel whatever emotions may arise.

Allow yourself to grieve

Ending your relationship with dieting can feel like a loss. After all, dieting has accompanied you through much of your life and provided a source of hope when things felt bleak. In our darkest moments, dieting promised that thinner, better days lay ahead. It symbolized a clear and simple path to improving our life (even if that path turned out to be paved with hot coals and shards of broken glass). This fantasy comforted us and served an important psychological purpose that we can honor, even if we are no longer dedicating ourselves to dieting. There is no one right way to feel during this process; try to allow space for whatever emotions may arise, including feelings of loss and grief, in this process of ending (or taking a break from) your relationship with dieting.

2

STEP 2: Challenge Your Assumptions about Weight and Health

"I don't want them to struggle with this the way that I have," Tracy told me tearfully in our initial session. A forty-two-year-old stay-at-home mom, Tracy had a life that revolved around her two children, Madison (age nine) and Liam (five). She was terrified of passing down her lifelong struggles with food and body image to her kids, just as she had inherited them from her own mother. She came to therapy determined to break the cycle.

Ever since she was born a big baby at 10 pounds 2 ounces, Tracy's weight had played a central role in her life. "You were so huge the doctor nearly dropped you," her mother laughed as she recounted her birth story in front of a group of Tracy's friends at her thirteenth birthday. Her mother wouldn't let her forget it for a second: Tracy was fat. Her mom was fat too, a fact that she tried to hide under oversized garments and suffocating girdles. In their small suburban town, Tracy's family seemed to have it all. High school sweethearts, her parents were well respected in the community. Her father was the pastor at the local church and her mother a teacher at the high school. Tracy's mother relished the perception of perfection and never wanted anyone to think that anything could be wrong. Having a fat daughter was a blemish on her well-manicured life. No matter how hard Tracy tried to win her over, nothing she did was ever good enough as long as she was in a fat body.

Family dinners were a source of humiliation and deprivation. Tracy ate special "dietetic" meals, portion-controlled plates that her mother weighed and measured to the exact specifications of whatever plan she was following at the moment. Meanwhile, her brother and father dined on grilled sirloin and mashed potatoes, spaghetti with Sunday sauce, or her mother's meat loaf with Ritz Crackers (always a crowd favorite). Her brother would mock her, sitting on the other side of the table and pinching his nose closed. "Pee-eww, your food smells like dog food, woof woof little doggie, eat your chow," he would say before putting his face to his plate on the table to mimic a dog eating. Her parents made only nominal efforts to intervene.

When Tracy was ten years old, she started sneaking downstairs late at night, after the rest of the family was asleep, to devour all the delicious food she wasn't allowed to eat. It was an adventure, scampering out of bed, remembering to avoid the floorboards that creaked so she didn't wake anyone up, and tiptoeing into the kitchen with her fuzzy bunny slippers and pink flashlight. She ate all the things that were forbidden and ate as much as she could while strategically leaving enough of each item that she wouldn't be found out. When her tummy simply couldn't hold anymore, she would slump back to bed, filled with anxiety that someone would discover her shameful secret.

It's been over twenty-five years since Tracy moved out from her parents' home, but she couldn't shake the old pattern of sneaking food. Each night, after her husband and kids were asleep, Tracy snuck into the kitchen and ate all the foods that she didn't allow herself to have during the day. In a day consumed with giving to others, this was time for herself. But while this way of eating satisfied a certain need, it also came with a tremendous amount of self-reproach, shame, and guilt. Plus, her kids were starting to notice.

"Mommy, where is the ice cream?" Liam had asked the previous week, after Tracy ate the pint of mint chocolate cookie dough that they had purchased on a recent grocery trip. How could she explain to her son that she had eaten all his precious ice cream? What would he think of her if he knew that she couldn't control her eating? "Um … I had to throw it away, honey, it had freezer burn," Tracy had lied. She couldn't even look him in the eye; she knew his disappointed expression all too well. Madison was starting to ask questions too, although slightly different from what her younger brother wanted to know. "Do I look fat?" she had asked that same week, pressing her unicorn and rainbow emblazoned dress against her round belly. Tracy's heart had leapt to her throat. She called me the next day to start treatment.

"I don't want my kids to know that their mom is fat," she stated in one of our early sessions. I looked at her, puzzled. Clearly, they saw her body. I asked her to explain more. "I don't want them to see me the way the world sees me. I don't want them to realize how disgusting I am. But they are getting older and they see. It's hard to hide anymore. I really just want to lose this weight."

Tracy described a recent family vacation to Walt Disney World, filled with what she described as one humiliating experience after another. "First there was the plane ride," she started off. "I see people's faces as I'm walking down the narrow aisle, their annoyance if I dare bump them as I come by, that look of dread, hoping I'm not coming to sit next to them. When we finally got to our seats, I realized with horror that the seat belt wouldn't buckle, and I needed the extender. I told the flight attendant *quietly*, I practically whispered it to her so that my kids didn't hear, and she nodded knowingly. Thankfully she was discreet about it, and Liam and Maddy were so engrossed in their iPads, I don't even think that they noticed. But I felt so ashamed. I tried to act like everything was normal, but my face turned so bright red I looked like Sebastian from *The Little Mermaid*.

"I can't say that the trip got much better from there. Once we got to Disney, the kids wanted me to go on the rides with them. I tried to pass it off to my husband, but they weren't having it. They wanted Mom. I was nervous that I wouldn't fit on the rides. Leading up to the trip, I read all the message boards and blogs about ride accessibility. I spent hours reading about every ride. Despite knowing that Disney is one of the most accommodating theme parks for people of size and having read stories of people bigger than me fitting on almost all the rides, I didn't feel reassured. All I could think about was holding up the whole line while I had to get off the ride and everyone laughing at me. The entire time we were waiting in line—and those are some long lines—my heart was pounding a million beats per minute. When we finally got to the front of the line, I shoved my body into the ride vehicle and prayed that the safety belt would close. Thankfully I fit, but if I keep gaining weight at this rate, I can't be sure that will be the case for next time. And then I slowed everyone down because I had to keep taking breaks with all the walking. My knees were killing me. Have you ever realized how huge Disney is? We were walking about ten miles each day, and my body just can't handle the extra weight. I thought about renting one of those electric scooters, but I just couldn't bring myself to do it. I need to lose this weight so I can feel better."

I asked Tracy about her knee pain. Was it typical for her to have pain when walking? She answered that it was, and that she was diagnosed several years ago with rheumatoid arthritis (RA), a disease with a strong genetic component that ran in her family along her father's bloodline. To my surprise, she didn't take any medication for the RA. Her doctor's only advice was to lose weight. I wondered why her doctor hadn't prescribed one of the medications shown in clinical trials to slow progression of RA symptoms when started early in treatment.[1] Was this recommendation to lose weight based on the doctor's weight bias instead of best practices in medicine? Would a thinner patient also have been recommended to lose weight? Or would they have been prescribed the medications shown in research to slow the disease progression?

A few weeks after our first meeting, Tracy started The Anti-Diet Plan group, where she met with Linda and the other group members. It didn't take long for her to discover that she wasn't alone in the mistreatment she received from medical doctors. Nearly every group participant who lived in a larger body had some experience of weight bias in the medical system. Linda's was particularly moving.

Seven years prior, cancer had invaded Linda's right breast. Her mother had died of breast cancer when Linda was twenty-four, and she had long feared that she would follow suit. *That's not how I'm going to go*, she firmly decided, as if it was all under her control. Like clockwork, each month, during her morning shower Linda would examine her breasts, searching and fearing that she would find something that wasn't supposed to be there. This monthly exam was one of the few times that Linda touched her own body. The thought of her squishy flesh disgusted her so much that even looking in the mirror was something to be avoided as much as possible. But she managed to make these breast exams such a detached clinical procedure that she hardly recognized the breasts under her hands as her own. One morning, when Linda was sixty-two years old, her nightmare came true. She felt a tiny lump toward the side of her right breast. Her heart beat faster as worst-case scenarios raced through her head. Images of her mother's final months came pouring back, how the disease had ravaged her body. She tried to push the thoughts away. It was so small, maybe it was nothing, she tried to reassure herself. But reassurance was hard to come by. Linda had been inordinately tired recently. She chalked it up to too many late nights out and didn't initially make much of it, but now, in context of the lump, it painted a terrifying picture. Linda made an appointment with her doctor as soon as she was out of the shower.

Less than a week later, Linda was sitting in the office of her internist. She hated going to the doctor. It seemed like no matter what was ailing her, the prescription was always the same. Lose weight. Each visit, she was reminded of all the ways her body wouldn't conform. Even the medical gown mocked her when the thin material resisted closing around her body. Her doctor, a trim young man in his forties, was a marathon runner. She knew this because he kept the medals displayed in his office, along with framed photographs of him crossing the finish line. "That was Boston," he said smugly as he caught Linda looking at one of the glass shadow boxes that held the mementos. "I twisted my ankle at mile 18, it hurt like hell, but I persisted onwards to finish the race. You know what they say, no pain, no gain, right? I ended up finishing with a decent time too," he said, with a chuckle. Linda smiled politely as she strategically held her gown closed to provide some modicum of coverage. Her doctor turned to the chart in front of him. "I see you've gained weight since the last time I saw you." He frowned. "Linda, we've talked about this before. You must get your weight under control. I want you to start exercising. Now, I know it's tough, but it's an important part of improving your health. You could try getting off the subway one stop early and walking a few blocks or take the stairs one flight instead of the elevator." A lifelong avid swimmer, Linda reminded him that she already exercised regularly. She had told him this at their last few visits too, when they had nearly identical conversations. *What's the point of him staring at that medical chart if he doesn't write down anything I say?* she wondered. "Ah okay, good for you. If you are already exercising, it's going to be a matter of diet then. Give the Whole30 a try. A lot of people are having success with that. Eliminate those carbohydrates. And sugar too. Let's follow up in three months and I want to see a lower weight, okay?" Linda nodded, feeling ashamed that she hadn't been able to stick to the same mandate after the last visit. He marked something down in the chart and turned to walk out of the room.

"Wait!" Linda called out with a panic. "The lump!" Her doctor turned back looking confused and walked back over to the chart. "Right, right, okay, let's give that a look." He put on cold latex gloves and hastily felt Linda's breast. "I don't feel anything," he said. "It was most likely just a fat deposit," he said. "Those can move around quite a bit and are common in people with, um, your body type." Back to the chart. "You just had a mammogram six months ago and it didn't show anything abnormal. I wouldn't worry about it. The low energy is probably just due to the excess weight. It's a big burden for your body to carry. A little exercise can help with that too. Let's focus on getting you active and following that diet plan, and I think you'll feel a lot better once you lose some weight. Now, I've got to get to my next patient. We'll meet again in a few months and I'm telling you, Linda, you'll notice a world of difference once you've dropped a few pounds."

Linda left the office feeling dejected. She went home and tried to feel for the lump again. It was tiny but definitely still there. Over the next few weeks, Linda tried unsuccessfully to put the lump out of her mind. But each morning, she felt her breast and confirmed the lump was still there.

Thankfully, she didn't wait too long before seeking a second opinion and getting the testing needed to diagnose stage 2 breast cancer.

"That's terrible," Tracy said, after hearing Linda's story. "I get the same lectures from my doctor too. It's why I avoid going to the doctor at all costs. I haven't been since my youngest was born. I mean, do I really need another lecture about my weight. Eat less? Exercise more? Thanks, Doc, I had never thought of that." She rolled her eyes.

In the scheme of things, Linda was lucky. She got the diagnosis and treatment that she needed with only a monthlong delay. Although in the world of cancer every single day counts, Linda survived her cancer and the course of her illness was not dramatically different due to her doctor's missed diagnosis. Unfortunately, the same can't be said for Ellen Maud Bennett, another fat woman, who was only a few years older than Linda when she got her cancer diagnosis at age sixty-four. She had suffered for years, feeling sick and seeking help from multiple doctors, before she was finally diagnosed with inoperable cancer mere days before her death. Her obituary, which went viral online, read in part: "A final message Ellen wanted to share was about the fat shaming she endured from the medical profession. Over the past few years of feeling unwell she sought out medical intervention and no one offered any support or suggestions beyond weight loss. Ellen's dying wish was that women of size make her death matter by advocating strongly for their health and not accepting that fat is the only relevant health issue."[2]

Weight Bias in the Medical System

I wish I could say that Ellen's or Linda's or Tracy's story was unique. They are not. Weight bias—defined as negative attitudes, beliefs, judgments, stereotypes, and discriminatory acts aimed at higher-weight individuals due to their weight—is ingrained in our medical system, just as it is ingrained into nearly every system in the US.

Doctors (along with family members) are the most common sources of weight stigma. Nearly 70 percent of women in larger bodies have experienced weight stigma at their doctor's office at least once, and more than half have experienced multiple stigmatizing experiences.[3] Most doctors hold negative attitudes about fat people, including beliefs that higher-weight patients are lazy, weak-willed, undisciplined, self-indulgent, and lacking in self-control.[4] Doctors characterize fat patients as awkward, unattractive, ugly, sloppy, dishonest, unintelligent, and unsuccessful; the heavier you are, the more likely you are to experience weight bias.[5] Not surprisingly, these negative attitudes affect the medical care that people in larger bodies receive.

Anti-fat attitudes are present from the early stages of medical training. Research suggests that nearly 70 percent of medical students hold preferences for thin people, 74 percent believe that "obesity" is caused by ignorance, and nearly 30 percent classified fat people as lazy.[6] Medical students who have themselves lost weight, particularly women, are the worst offenders.[7] Derogatory humor at the expense of fat people is commonplace in medical training and reflects students' (and their teachers') disdain of fat bodies, the belief that fat patients are to blame for their medical conditions, and the feeling that fat patients cause extra work.[8]

Despite all the evidence to the contrary (remember what we learned about set point theory in chapter 1?), most doctors incorrectly believe that weight is a matter of choice and personal responsibility. Doctors most commonly cite diet and exercise as the causes of "obesity" and believe that a lack of motivation in these areas is the reason patients don't lose weight.[9] These inaccurate beliefs play a key role in perpetuating weight stigma. If doctors believe that people can simply *choose* to be thinner (after all, it's just a matter of eating less and exercising more, right?), that must mean that fat people aren't making the right choices. And probably they aren't making the right choices because they are lazy, lack motivation and discipline, don't care about their health, or are just too stupid. This leads doctors to blame their fat patients for any health issues that may arise. *Why should I have to spend my time dealing with this patient's health problems when this could all be solved by them getting off the couch and putting away the bag of chips? They aren't even doing anything to help themselves. If they don't care about their health, why should I?*

In research studies, doctors report less desire to help fat patients. Seeing them as a burden, they feel more frustration, have less patience, show less respect, and have more annoyance for higher-weight patients. They even report liking their job less when they interact with fat patients. Because doctors believe that fat patients don't take care of themselves and will not comply with medical recommendations anyway, they spend less time in visits (one study suggests nearly 30 percent less time) and provide less education about health conditions and treatment. Doctors view their visits with fat patients as a waste of time.[10]

This pervasive weight bias means fat people receive subpar medical care and have subsequently worse health outcomes. Higher-weight patients are nearly three times as likely as smaller-bodied patients to report that they have been denied appropriate medical care.[11] It is not uncommon for patients to be denied access to surgery due to their body size. Doctors are more reluctant to perform preventative screening procedures (such as a pelvic exam).[12] Even when willing, doctors often lack the training and proper equipment to adequately care for their larger-bodied patients.

Fat patients are commonly prescribed weight loss instead of more effective evidence-based treatments for their symptoms. This means that while patients are spinning their wheels trying to lose weight, medical problems are not being effectively treated and can worsen over time. By the time that correct diagnoses are made and/or treatments administered, illnesses are further progressed and often more difficult to treat, with poorer prognoses. One study of medical students showed that only 5 percent of doctors-to-be prescribed medication to a patient complaining of difficulty breathing when the patient was described as "obese," compared with 23 percent who prescribed medication when the patient was described as "normal weight" *with the exact same symptoms.*[13] Instead of being prescribed medications proven to improve shortness of breath, the fat patients were prescribed "lifestyle changes," otherwise known as weight loss.

Fat patients are less likely to receive "patient-centered care," a method of medical treatment described in the *New England Journal of Medicine* as when "an individual's specific health needs and desired health outcomes are the driving force behind all health care decisions and quality measurements."[14] This is considered the gold standard of medical care and is associated with improved health outcomes for people who have the privilege of receiving it.[15]

The awful stigmatizing encounters that fat people have with health care professionals make them avoid the doctor. Research suggests that higher-weight patients are likely to delay or forgo essential preventative care, such as routine screenings for cancer prevention (including age-appropriate screenings for breast, cervical, and colorectal cancer).[16] When asked why they are delaying or forgoing health care, their overwhelming response was weight bias. In one study that asked women about barriers to routine gynecological cancer screenings, 68 percent of "obese" women reported that they delayed seeking health care because of their weight, and 83 percent reported that their weight was a barrier to getting appropriate health care.[17] Participants described worry about or past experiences of disrespectful treatment and negative attitudes from health care providers, embarrassment about being weighed, receiving unsolicited advice to lose weight, and gowns, exam tables, and other equipment being too small to be functional. The percentage of women reporting these concerns increased as BMI increased. They were less likely to receive timely screenings despite feeling "moderately" or "very concerned" about cancer symptoms (so it's not that they just didn't care about their health). Similarly, other studies report women avoiding health care because of having gained weight, not wanting to be weighed, not wanting to undress in the exam room, knowing they would be told to lose weight, and feeling embarrassment or discomfort.[18]

If you live in a larger body, you likely have experienced weight stigma in health care settings. You may have even blamed your own body for the treatment you received. We are taught to trust our doctors and believe that they have our best interest at heart. If we felt slighted, it must've been in our head. If our doctor told us that our symptoms will improve with weight loss, there must be science behind that recommendation. If they told us that a certain diet plan works well, it must be our fault if we can't stick to it. It's an odd plot twist when we are blamed for the very health problems being exacerbated by weight stigma. As we are about to learn, it is likely that pervasive weight stigma plays a substantial role in many of the health issues commonly blamed on "obesity."

The Effect of Weight Stigma on Your Health

Unless you have been living under a rock for the past few decades, you've probably heard the messages that "obesity" is bad for your health. Public health campaigns warn of the risks of fatness, linking higher weight to everything from cancer to diabetes to heart disease to depression to early death. The media would have us believe that our weight is directly responsible for these health issues. If we look at the research, however, the relationship is far less clear than what the general public believes. Does being at a higher weight cause health problems? Or could there be other factors that occur alongside fatness—such as weight stigma—that help explain the association?

Unfortunately, many of the large-scale studies that find an association between weight and disease do not account for important confounding variables (also called mediating variables) that influence the relationship between weight and health. In research, a confounding variable can make it appear that two variables are related, when in fact a third variable is responsible for the relationship. Here is an example: There is a strong association between increased ice cream consumption and murders. If we only look at those two data points and try to infer a relationship between them, we may conclude that ice cream turns people into violent killers (and with all the hype around sugar, I wouldn't be surprised if this argument has been made!). But if you have ever taken any introductory statistics class, you may remember the refrain "correlation is not causation," and this is exactly what it is talking about. There is another variable that occurs alongside ice cream consumption and murders that better explains the relationship. Can you guess it? Warm weather. A lot of research documents higher homicide rates in the summer when people are more likely to be out and about, doing things like buying ice cream and killing people.

So, what are the confounding variables that often get left out of weight research? There are a bunch, but I'm going to run through a few that I think are most important and summarize some of the research that has taken the complexities of these relationships into account. The variables that I want to talk about here are weight stigma, internalized weight bias, health behaviors including nutrition and fitness, socioeconomic status, and race. Many of these intersect with each other, creating multilayered determinants of health, so keep that in mind as you read.

Research suggests that weight stigma is associated with a 60 percent increased risk of death, independent of BMI.[19] We just learned a lot about weight stigma in medical settings and how this can lead to missed diagnoses, delayed treatments, avoidance of medical care, and lower rates of preventative screenings. "Obesity" is often referred to as the "leading preventable cause of cancer." But people at higher weights are less likely to have regular age-appropriate cancer screenings due to weight stigma. Doctors are more reluctant to perform procedures like pelvic exams on larger-bodied patients. Medical professionals often lack the equipment necessary to adequately examine, screen, and diagnose fat patients. For example, many diagnostic imaging facilities do not have MRI scanners that accommodate larger bodies. Doctors, who have typically been trained in treating only thin bodies, report more difficulty doing screening procedures with larger-bodied people. This leads to missed diagnoses, delays in treatment, and worse prognoses. One study estimates that preventative screening reduces the risk of dying from cancer by 25–30 percent.[20] It's no wonder "obesity" is a risk factor for cancer—fat people aren't getting the same level of preventive care as thinner people. Is it fatness that is a risk for cancer? Or the lack of preventive screening procedures?

Weight stigma also underlies many of the mental health issues associated with "obesity." Studies suggest that weight stigma, rather than weight, is related to mood disorders, such as depression and anxiety.[21] Experiences of weight stigma are positively associated with depression, above and beyond the effect of BMI.[22] In particular, the experience of being teased about your weight plays a key role in both depression and low self-esteem. A 2003 research study suggests that weight-based teasing explains the relationship between "obesity" and depression.[23] Weight stigma also explains the relationship between "obesity" and low self-esteem, lack of self-acceptance, lack of self-compassion, and poor body image.[24] It seems as though it is not the weight in and of itself that causes emotional distress as much as the interpersonal mistreatment that people endure because of their weight.

Internalized weight bias, a phenomenon where people turn weight-based societal scorn and devaluation inward and apply these negative stereotypes to themselves, is associated with poor health outcomes.[25] A 2017 study by Rebecca Pearl and her colleagues examined the role of internalized weight stigma in the relationship between BMI and metabolic syndrome, the name for a cluster of risk factors for cardiometabolic disease and type 2 diabetes that is commonly associated with "obesity."[26] They found that, after controlling for the possible confounding effect of BMI and other variables, participants who scored high on a measure of weight bias internalization had three times greater odds of meeting criteria for metabolic syndrome and six times greater odds of having high triglycerides (fat in your blood that can increase risk of heart disease) and/or taking medication for dyslipidemia (i.e., high cholesterol) than participants who had low weight bias internalization. Weight bias internalization is higher in people who are dieting and trying to lose weight than in the general population.[27] This makes a lot of sense—people with high internalized weight bias feel that their body is bad and are desperate to change it so are more likely to try dieting to lose weight. In addition to increasing the risk of health outcomes like metabolic disease, internalized weight bias is linked with psychological outcomes including reduced quality of life, poorer psychological functioning, disordered eating, decreased ability to self-regulate food intake, and avoidance of exercise. It's a vicious cycle where we blame our body, thinking that if we just lost weight we would feel better emotionally and physically. But these thoughts stem from weight bias—the very same system that is making us sick!

People living in larger bodies face discrimination and bias in almost every aspect of life, with severity of discrimination increasing along with

BMI.[28] Interpersonally people in larger bodies are commonly bullied, harassed, and teased by family members, peers, and strangers. This may include receiving a nasty glare when you go to sit next to someone on the subway, hearing someone making animal sounds at you from a passing car window, scrolling through dating sites and seeing profiles that request "no fatties please," or being sexually objectified and degraded by potential romantic partners. Living in a larger body means being uncertain if you can fit when you dine out, go to the theater, fly on an airplane, or go on an amusement park ride. It's being harassed on social media for posting the same pictures thinner people are applauded for posting—enjoying summer in a bathing suit, eating delicious food, or just going about your daily life.

In educational settings, higher-weight female students are only half as likely to attend college when compared with smaller-bodied peers. Teachers commonly exhibit anti-fat bias, leading to inferior treatment of fat students, which affects academic achievement. Bullying from peers also impacts achievement. Students with a BMI in the "obese" range have lower academic achievement than lower-weight peers. Weight-based discrimination continues in employment settings, with disadvantages in hiring, wages, promotions, and termination. In experiments when employers were shown two job candidates with the exact same qualifications except one candidate was "overweight" and one was not, employers viewed the "overweight" applicant more negatively and were less likely to want to hire them. People with a BMI in the "severely obese" category were 100 times more likely to experience employment discrimination than someone whose BMI is in the "normal" range. White women with a BMI in the "severely obese" category are paid 24 percent less than white women with a BMI in the "normal" range. Black women, already subject to a wage penalty due to racism, are penalized again if they are fat; Black women with a BMI in the "severely obese" category are paid 14.6 percent less than their thinner Black female colleagues.[29]

Weight stigma affects our health through stress responses in our body. Studies have demonstrated heightened physiological reactivity in response to experiences of weight stigmatization, including heightened cortisol (referred to as the "stress hormone") reactivity, C-reactive protein (a marker of inflammation), and blood pressure (which can rise under stress).[30] Chronic stress, a natural response to living in a stigmatized body—one that's deemed unacceptable by society (weight bias) and by ourselves (internalized weight bias)—leads to oxidative stress and cortisol secretion, both implicated in metabolic syndrome.

Weight-based discrimination—especially in educational and employment settings—also impacts income, which is one of the most well-documented predictors of health. In the US, as BMI increases, income decreases. And as income decreases, so does life expectancy. Of all the social determinants of health, income is the most influential. Research indicates that the gap in life expectancy between the richest 1 percent and the poorest 1 percent of people in the US was more than fourteen years for men and ten years for women.[31] These health discrepancies occur across the income spectrum; no matter how much money you earn, the more money you make, the lower your likelihood of disease and premature death. There are many reasons why income has such an extreme impact on health—including but not limited to the chronic stress of financial instability, access to health care, access to fresh fruits and vegetables, food insecurity, availability of time and places to be physically active, and environmental pollution. Black, Indigenous, and People of Color (BIPOC) populations who are classified as "obese" face multiple layers of oppression through both weight-based discrimination and racism, which also impacts income, wealth, and health. Additional layers of oppression lead to worse health outcomes; for example, fat Black people with a disability (who face weight bias, racism, and ableism) confront more barriers than fat Black people who are able-bodied.

Due to the pervasive weight bias discussed earlier, most fat people have tried to lose weight at one time or another. It's only natural that people seek to escape a stigmatized condition, right? And we already learned in chapter 1 that the most likely outcome of dieting and other methods of intentional weight loss is weight cycling, where a person initially loses weight and then regains it over time. While the research on the health impact of weight cycling has mixed results, there is evidence to suggest that weight cycling may increase the risk of certain health conditions commonly associated with "obesity." Studies have shown a link between weight cycling and increased risk of cardiovascular disease, heart attack and stroke, type 2 diabetes, metabolic syndrome, hypertension, cancer, bone fractures, and increased risk of death.[32] In older adults weight cycling is associated with impaired ability to engage in daily activities, limited mobility, and increased risk of death.[33] A 2019 study found that weight cycling is associated with a 50 percent increase in risk of death, even when controlling for other cardiovascular risk factors and body weight.[34] In addition to the dangerous physiological risks, weight cycling also takes a toll on our mental well-being. It is associated with increased risk of eating disorders, psychopathology (including anxiety and depression), and life dissatisfaction.[35] Experts believe that the process of weight cycling elicits an inflammatory response in the body that is associated with negative health outcomes.[36] Perhaps not coincidentally, "obesity" is also thought to cause health problems through a similar inflammatory process in our body, which again raises the questions: What is really making us sick? Is it our weight or is it weight cycling?

The relationship between weight and health is complex. When we believe that weight loss will improve our health, we ignore all the other factors that impact our well-being. When we focus on weight loss as the path to health, we embody biased beliefs that our weight is under our control and is just a matter of motivation and willpower. Conversely if we don't lose weight it's because we are lazy, have no self-control, and are bad. Ironically it is these very beliefs (i.e., internalized weight bias) that are making us sick.

And even if being at a higher weight *is* associated with health problems, we know that long-term weight loss is unsustainable and that dieting is associated with a host of health issues including weight cycling, increased internalized weight bias, increased inflammation, and increased risk of eating disorders, disordered eating, and body image dissatisfaction. The good news is that there is lots you can do to improve your health without focusing on weight loss or dieting. We'll explore that later in this chapter.

Where Does Weight Stigma Stem From?

The "American Dream" emphasizes personal responsibility and self-determination. Our "pull yourself up by your bootstraps" ethos teaches us that anyone can succeed if they just try hard enough. We love feel-good stories of people who found a way to rise up from dire circumstances. These narratives reassure those with privilege that they have earned their place in the world; *I'm successful because I've worked hard and those who are less fortunate just aren't trying as hard as I am.* It also leads people in marginalized groups to blame themselves for their hardships; *if that person was able to rise up, what's wrong with me that I'm having such a hard time?* It ignores the systemic barriers that marginalized people face, and it discounts the doors that swing open for privileged people as they move through the world. In this myth of personal responsibility and meritocracy, fatness becomes a choice. Fat people aren't working hard enough to be thin. They are lazy, gluttonous, and slovenly. In our puritanical culture that values hard work and discipline, fatness is evidence of moral inferiority. The irony, of course, is that weight is definitely not under our control (as we learned in chapter 1). When we think about how miserable diet culture makes life for fat people and the desperate and dramatic measures so many people take to lose weight, it's clear that few people would choose to be fat. Not because there is anything inherently wrong with being fat. But because being fat in a culture that hates fat people is pretty rough.

Why did fatness become stigmatized in the first place? Fatphobia is inextricably linked with racism, as Sabrina Strings explains in her book *Fearing the Black Body*.[37] The origins of fatphobia can be traced back to the transatlantic slave trade and "race science," a system to classify races as superior and inferior. White people, who created the categories of race science, conveniently put themselves at the top of the hierarchy. To rationalize the kidnapping and enslavement of Black people, Africans were categorized as an inferior race. While skin color was initially used to differentiate the races, interracial sex (including rape of Black enslaved women by white male slaveholders) in the colonies made skin color a less reliable indicator. Additional characteristics were needed to categorize the races, and body size became a prominent one. Blackness was associated with a "robust" body size, especially for women, which was said to stem from uncontrolled "animal instincts" of excessive eating, drinking, and sex. To differentiate themselves, in the late eighteenth century white people started to embrace a thin ideal that also embodied the Protestant ethics of self-control and restraint. Prior to this time, the beauty ideal in the US was of a larger woman. Fatness was associated with wealth and good health, while thinness was associated with illness and frailty. By the end of the nineteenth century, however, fatness was firmly associated with immorality and racial inferiority. Thinness became a sign of white American exceptionalism, proving that white people had more self-discipline than the unruly African people they had enslaved.

While race science was evolving, Protestant ideas were also gaining popularity. Protestants believed that hard work and self-discipline were the path to salvation (not unlike the "pull yourself up by the bootstraps" ethos of the modern US). Moderation, self-control, and restraint were virtues associated with thinness (and whiteness). Fatness (and Blackness) became associated with laziness, lack of discipline, gluttony, and overindulgence. Weight loss was a godly virtuous pursuit. This association of body size and morality continues to prevail in modern society.

Science supported these prevailing cultural norms around race with the development of fields like anthropometry and craniometry, which sought to identify physical differences between races and create hierarchical classifications. The BMI was developed as part of this "science." In the 1830s Belgian academic Lambert Adolphe Jacques Quetelet developed "the Quetelet Method" to study white western European men's bodies, which he considered to be ideal. It wasn't until more than 100 years later, in 1972, that the Quetelet Method was adapted and renamed the body mass index (BMI) by Ancel Keys (remember him from the Minnesota Starvation Study in chapter 1?). Like Quetelet, Keys only used data from white Anglo-Saxon populations to develop and norm the BMI. In 1985 the National Institutes of Health (NIH) took this formula designed as a statistical tool to measure a white population and started using BMI to define "obesity" on an individual level.

BMI has always been a lousy measure of health. The Centers for Disease Control and Prevention (CDC) cautions that BMI does not distinguish between fat, muscle, bone density, and fat distribution.[38] BMI consistently overestimates risks for certain racial groups, particularly Black people, and underestimates the risks for other groups, like Asian people. Even among "obesity" researchers who are dedicated to the weight-normative (i.e., fat is bad) perspective, the BMI is widely recognized as inaccurate. Yet it remains the most commonly used measure to assess health.

In 1998 the NIH decided to lower the BMI cutoff to be classified as "overweight," shifting 29 million people from "healthy" to "overweight" overnight. This decision was made in concert with the International Obesity Task Force, an organization funded by pharmaceutical drug companies that manufacture weight loss drugs.[39] The chairman of the NIH committee in charge of the decision to lower the BMI criteria was a consultant to several drug manufacturers and on the advisory board of Weight Watchers.[40] How convenient that lowering the BMI threshold meant that 29 million people would suddenly be in the market for the weight loss pills and diet plans that would financially benefit the people who lowered the threshold.

A similar decision was made in 2013, when the American Medical Association (AMA) classified "obesity" as a disease. In considering this decision, the AMA convened with the American Council on Science and Public Health, a committee of appointed AMA members who studied the issue for more than a year. The council concluded that "obesity" should not be classified as a disease. In their report, they stated the flawed nature of BMI and the fact that some people with "obesity" do not experience elevated health risk and some, in fact, demonstrate protective factors (termed "the obesity paradox").[41] It was a highly unusual move for the AMA to go against the recommendations of their own advisory board. As reported in the *New York Times*, the AMA rejected the findings of their board and decided to move forward, passing the resolution to classify "obesity" as a disease.[42] The resolution was introduced and pushed forward in part by the American Association of Clinical Endocrinologists (AACE), an organization with close ties to the pharmaceutical and bariatric-surgery industries.[43] In a local meeting of the American Society for Metabolic and Bariatric Surgery that I attended, during the presidential address the chapter president formally thanked their friends at AACE for pushing the resolution through—presumably since for obvious reasons it looked better for AACE (an organization that, to the public, would appear to have less obvious financial investment in the resolution) to be behind it instead of their own group. The decision also coincided with the release of two new FDA-approved weight loss drugs, the first new ones brought to market in over a decade. Both the pharmaceutical and bariatric-surgery industries benefited greatly by the AMA's classification of obesity as a disease because it expanded insurance coverage for bariatric surgery and weight loss drugs. It also encouraged doctors to recommend surgery and weight loss medications for their higher-weight patients because, after all, now "obesity" was a disease and diseases need treatment. The AMA decision was followed by marketing efforts like the "Treat Obesity Seriously" campaign by the Obesity Society (another professional organization with ties to the food, pharmaceutical, and bariatric-surgery industries) aimed at "educating" clinicians about "obesity" treatments (namely surgery and medications).

The medical, pharmaceutical, and weight loss industries are tied together by a string of financial entanglements. In 2015 the Endocrine Society, a "global community of physicians and scientists dedicated to accelerating scientific breakthroughs and improving patient health and well being" (per their home page at www.endocrine.org), released guidelines on the treatment of obesity. These guidelines promote the use of new and expensive weight loss medications.[44] Unsurprisingly, the lead author has received payment from all the pharmaceutical companies that manufacture the medications recommended in the guidelines.[45] Even some organizations dedicating to eradicating weight stigma are just shells for the weight loss industry. For example, the Obesity Action Coalition is funded by the pharmaceutical company Novo Nordisk (which makes drugs being studied for weight loss), the American Society for Metabolic and Bariatric Surgery (a professional organization for bariatric surgeons), Bariatric Advantage (a company that makes vitamins and supplements for people who undergo bariatric surgery), and Potomac Currents (a lobbying group whose clients include both the American Society for Metabolic and Bariatric Surgery and the Obesity Action Coalition).[46] Rather than truly fight weight bias, this organization centers its main activities around increasing access to weight loss drugs and weight loss surgery.

It is not uncommon for "obesity" researchers, leaders of professional organizations, and policy makers to be on the payroll of the pharmaceutical, diet, and weight loss industries. This makes it nearly impossible for anyone—from well-educated physicians to the average citizen trying to make informed decisions about health—to know where their "scientific" or "medical" information is truly coming from. Are health guidelines designed to improve our health, or are they designed to turn a profit for the weight loss industry?

How Can We Improve Our Health without Dieting or Weight Loss?

Dieting and hating yourself isn't working. In fact, it's pretty darned harmful. But you didn't need me to tell you that, did you? It echoes what we deeply know through our own lived experiences. The good news is that there is another way! We don't need to live our life on pause, waiting until the scale hits some magical number to feel better. Much of what we seek through weight loss is available to us right now, at this very moment. If you have been dieting or trying to lose weight as a means of improving your health, you may be relieved to know that there are behaviors that we can engage in to improve our health that have absolutely nothing to do with losing weight.

When I talk about "improving health," I want to highlight that health is going to look different for everyone. Our bodies are individual, unique, ever-changing beings. Some of us are living with chronic medical issues that will always be a part of our life in one way or another. Some of us don't have access to everything that we need to feel as good as we can in our bodies. And for some of us, reaching that optimal level of personal wellness just isn't our number one priority. That's all okay. We are not morally obligated to improve our health. If you are living in a larger body, you may have felt compelled to "prove" your health (whether through performing "healthy" behaviors like ordering a salad when you go out to eat or by sharing details of your health history with people) because, as much as diet culture hates fat people, it really hates sick fat people. Health becomes a lifeline for fat people to justify their existence. *I'm not a burden on the system, I don't have any health problems. I exercise regularly. I eat healthy.* As if this is the response needed to fatphobia. *Hate other fat people, the sick ones, those are the bad fat people. I'm okay.* It is human nature to want to differentiate ourselves from a stigmatized group, even for people within that group. Health has become a yardstick to measure acceptability of fatness. It is essential that we always remember—healthy or unhealthy, thin or fat, young or old—the problem is not your body. I'll say it again and again in this book and I still won't have said it enough. The problem is not your body. The problem is weight stigma. The problem is fatphobia. The problem is racism. The problem is diet culture. You are deserving of respect and compassion because you are a human being, not because of your health status.

Increasing health-promoting behaviors in gentle and compassionate ways can improve your health completely independent of dieting or losing weight. Which makes sense, right? Health behaviors improve our health—it's not rocket science. But diet culture obscures our view of what is right in front of us.

Four healthy behaviors are consistently associated with health regardless of BMI: not smoking, not drinking alcohol to excess, eating fruits and vegetables, and being physically active. A 2008 study looking at over 20,000 people found that increasing these four behaviors could increase life expectancy by as much as fourteen years, regardless of BMI.[47] Similarly a large 2012 study found that these same four healthy behaviors were associated with improved health and decreased mortality regardless of BMI.[48] There is a large body of research suggesting that fitness has a far larger impact on health than BMI. A review paper that analyzed results of ten studies found that fit people with a BMI in the "overweight" or "obese" categories had similar mortality risks to fit people with a BMI in the "normal" range.[49] Another review found fit individuals with a BMI in the "obese" range had lower risk of death than unfit individuals who had a BMI in the "normal" range.[50] When it comes to our health, fitness seems to play a far larger role than weight. Other behaviors associated with improved health are managing stress and getting enough sleep—and both can be improved with meditation, which we'll be learning about in the next chapter.

The problem is health behaviors are typically couched in a weight loss framework. "Wellness" has become a code word for "thin" (and "wealthy"— most of these products and services are out of reach for all but the upper classes). "Health" has become another way to deride fat people's bodies, claiming that it is unhealthy to be fat and that is a reason to harass, bully, and otherwise mistreat people in larger bodies. Yet the same people who are so concerned about fat people's health rarely voice concern when they see thinner people engaging in similar behaviors. For example, a thin person who posts a picture on social media eating fast food is celebrated for being "brave" and rejecting diet culture, whereas a fat person who posts a picture of themselves eating the same foods is berated for "glorifying obesity." At the end of the day, it's not really about health; it's about body size and shape. In this context, we only think that health behaviors are valuable if they result in weight loss and a closer approximation of the beauty ideal. We often engage in these behaviors, like exercising or eating more fruits and vegetables, when we embark on a new weight loss plan and then abandon them as soon as we stop seeing the results we want. When viewed through a weight loss lens, these health-promoting behaviors become punitive; *I must go to the gym because my body is bad. I have to eat this sad salad instead of that delicious burger because it's on my diet plan.* They feed into our internalized weight bias (e.g., *I can't believe I caved and had the burger, I'm such a failure, I'll have to work out twice as much this week or this is going straight to my hips!*) and keep us stuck on the diet–overeating–self-hatred roller coaster. But when we can truly separate out health from weight loss and approach our well-being from a place of compassion instead of self-hatred, we are able to engage in behaviors in a totally different way. We'll be learning more about how to do this in the following chapters, but you've already started making these changes! Understanding that diets don't work, that weight loss isn't sustainable, and that our weight doesn't determine our health helps us unlearn the internalized weight stigma that is negatively impacting our health. It helps free us from diet culture and creates the space for us to listen to what our body truly needs.

Takeaways

We have covered a lot of ground in this chapter and I want to wrap it up with a few takeaway points. One of the biggest objections I hear to letting go of dieting and weight loss goals is: *But what about my health? I have health issues that would improve if I lost weight.* Here is what we know. The relationship between weight and health is complex and far muddier than the evening news would have us believe. Weight-based discrimination and stigma, weight cycling, health behaviors, income, and race play large roles in the association between weight and health. And even if being at a higher weight *is* associated with increased risk of health problems, we must remember that we have no good way to help people lose and maintain significant weight long-term. Dieting is not effective and can be dangerous. It increases internalized weight bias, weight cycling, body image dissatisfaction, risk of eating disorders and disordered eating, and other health problems. Dieting is associated with many of the very same health problems we are seeking to improve through weight loss.

We have far more effective ways for improving health. Research shows that focusing on four health-promoting behaviors—eating more fruits and vegetables, being physically active, not smoking, and not drinking alcohol in excess—improves health completely independent of weight. If we want to improve our health, let's focus on behaviors that promote our well-being, not weight loss.

TAKE-ACTION ACTIVITIES

Update your reasons list

Remember the list from chapter 1 that you made of the reasons you want to lose weight? Take another look at that list and identify if anything has changed based on what you learned in this chapter. Anything that you connected to weight loss before that you can separate now?

Let's make some goals!

What is one thing that you want to work on now, at your current body size? Is there something that you previously connected to needing to lose weight that you can start working on now? It can be about health, mental well-being, relationships, or anything else! What action steps can you take to start working toward this goal?

The SMART framework can be helpful for goal setting. SMART goals are

- Specific: Try to clearly define your goal; don't make it too broad or general.

- Measurable: How will you quantify your goal? How will you measure your progress?

- Achievable: Make your goal something you can realistically attain.

- Relevant: Pick a goal that matters to you; think about your *why*.

- Time-Specific: Set a realistic timeline (I recommend a timeline that will be after you've finished reading this book, so you can use all the tools).

3

STEP 3: Learn the Five-Minute Meditation

Mia came rushing into my office five minutes after the first session of The Anti-Diet Plan group started. "I'm so sorry I'm late, the train took forever," she said as she frantically stripped off layers of winter gear. It was a particularly cold February night in New York City, but her face was flushed and sweaty under her furry winter hat, scarf, and oversized jacket. This is always a hazard in New York winters—it's freezing outside but the subways are heated, and you can really work up a sweat all layered up rushing from one place to another. As she peeled off her outerwear, I saw Mia was wearing an oversized green sweater woven with silver thread over shiny black leggings with the knee-high boots that were in style that year. Those boots were nearly impossible to find in plus fashion (something many of my clients lamented that season); it was as if footwear designers had forgotten to account for varying calf sizes. But that wasn't something Mia had to worry about, as her body (including her calves) fit into "straight size" (non-plus-size) clothing, albeit the upper sizes. Despite this thin privilege, Mia was convinced that her body was too large, especially compared to her coworkers who looked like they had just stepped off the fashion runway.

Mia hung her bag on a hook by the door and sat down in an empty seat on the couch next to Linda. She pulled her body in tight, trying to make herself as small as possible, lest she infringe on Linda's space. She tugged on the neck of her heavy sweater, droplets of sweat still rolling down her brow. "Take a load off," Linda said, patting the space on the couch next to her. "I won't bite. Make yourself comfortable." Mia smiled politely but her body didn't ease up. Despite clearly overheating, she clutched her jacket like a toddler's security blanket on her lap, covering her body.

The group members went around the circle, introducing themselves and sharing what they hoped to get from the group. Linda focused on her health concerns and difficulties with aging. Tracy talked about her longing to set a healthier example for her children. Michael (who you'll meet in chapter 5) wanted to stop thinking about food all the time. When it was Mia's turn, she said, "I'm stuck in this love-hate relationship with food. Sometimes it doesn't really matter to me, I can go all day without eating, especially when I'm busy at work, but when I come home, it's like a switch flips and all I can think about is ordering a ton of food. Every night I try to talk myself out of doing it, just go to the grocery store and cook something at home, but then I'm so tired and I think about what a crappy day I've had and I say, you know what, you deserve this, after all you've been through, you deserve to have a little treat. So I order takeout, sometimes two or three or four dishes, and I eat it all. Then I get terrible stomachaches and I'm like, ugh, why did I do that? Why can't I just control myself?" The other group members nodded empathetically. This struggle was one many could relate to.

Mia believed her issues with food stemmed from a lack of self-control. She saw the problem as overeating and believed that if only she could be more disciplined, she could avoid these problematic episodes. When she would go long stretches without eating, Mia felt accomplished. After all, she was eating so much in the evening, if she could go most of the earlier part of the day without eating, surely this would help balance things out? Mia felt disconnected from her body. She kept herself so busy and distracted that she couldn't hear her internal cues like hunger or fullness until they were screaming for her attention and she had no choice but listen. By this time, her hunger felt overwhelming and out of control.

Mia was always on the go. She had moved to "the city" three years prior to take her dream job working with a well-known fashion designer. As a junior assistant, her job was demanding. Her day started at 9 a.m. when she had to have her boss's skinny vanilla latte waiting hot at his desk. She then spent the next ten to twelve hours shuffling around doing whatever urgent task of the day needed to be done. Drop samples at the *Vogue* office? Sure thing. Bring Fluffy to the groomers? No problem, Boss. Arrange for a dinner party for thirty guests that evening? Right on top of it. Everyone else at her office seemed to be the perfect vision of New York style. They wore the latest fashions, ate the same salad from the overpriced salad shop around the corner, and worked out at the trendy boutique fitness studio that Gwyneth Paltrow was rumored to frequent (although no one had actually ever seen her there). Mia simultaneously hated and envied them. They were all extraordinarily thin, and gaining weight seemed to be their greatest fear. Looking like Mia was their greatest fear.

Mia was the odd one out at work. While she had a cordial relationship with her coworkers, she felt intensely uncomfortable. In her head she couldn't stop comparing herself to them. She always came out on the losing end of these comparisons. Whatever she wore was too frumpy, whatever she ate wasn't "healthy" enough, and her body was wrong in every way imaginable. She felt isolated and lonely.

The last thing that Mia wanted to do was be present with herself. The busyness at work was a welcome distraction from her inner thoughts. When she wasn't preoccupied with work, she filled the space in her mind with podcasts and music, streaming through the earbuds that were practically implanted into her ears. She tried to eat "healthy" (read: diet) but broke her own rules more often than not. For most of the day food was an afterthought; she would grab what she could when she could, often going long periods of time without eating and then eating foods that she judged as "bad" because they were quick, readily available, and she was hungry. In the evenings she "treated" herself after a hard day with takeout from local restaurants. One of the greatest things about Manhattan is that you can have anything delivered at any moment. If she didn't have a full multicourse meal it felt like a deprivation. But after eating her meals, Mia didn't feel good. She suffered stomachaches almost every night, ending her day doubled over in bed, wondering why she had done this to herself yet again.

Diet culture makes us feel conflicted about food. For Mia, this manifested in a "checking out" or disconnection from her body. She subsisted on coffee for most of the morning and then didn't eat anything until midafternoon. By the time that she forced herself to stop for lunch, her hunger had reached a fever pitch that was hard to ignore. Then she would think about what to eat. She would tell herself that she should eat a salad, like her coworkers did. But this never seemed appealing, plus it was so expensive. She was the most junior and lowest-paid employee at the office, and unlike her coworkers who didn't seem to think twice about spending $20 on a salad or $50 on a fitness class, Mia was trying to survive on a single income in one of the most expensive cities in the world. So she would often go to the deli on the corner where they made cheap, delicious, and filling chicken parmesan sandwiches, or grab a couple slices of pizza from her local $1 slice spot, or just find whatever else was fast and convenient. She judged these choices, berating herself for not picking a "healthier" option. Immersed in conflict, self-hatred, and extreme hunger, she ate the food quickly, not really tasting it and giving little thought to what she was in the mood to eat or when she felt comfortably full. Having now "blown it," Mia would soon start fantasizing about dinner. What should I get tonight? Maybe dim sum from Wo Hop (one of the oldest—and arguably the best—Chinese restaurants in Chinatown)? Or spaghetti al limone from Supper? A sub from the Meatball Shop? She would go back and forth in her mind for hours, trying to settle on the perfect meal.

When she finally got her food, she would bring it into her bedroom and eat it while zoning out to the TV. She ate until she was stuffed, and felt tired and sick afterward. She berated herself mercilessly, telling herself things that she would never dream of saying to anyone else. She searched for distractions to get her away from her body and her harsh inner voice.

Sometimes this was binge-watching Netflix or listening to podcasts or getting swept up in work emails. Between these distractions at home and her chronic busyness at work, there were very few moments of being present with her eating experiences or being aware of the signals that her body was sending her at any given moment.

Back in the group session, I started talking about mindfulness. Mia rolled her eyes. "Looks like you have some feelings about that," I said, with a smile.

"It's just that I've tried mindfulness before, they always do it at the end of yoga class, and I can't stand it. My mind doesn't stay still." This is one of the most common misperceptions of mindfulness—that it's about quieting your mind. People often think that they aren't meditating correctly if they aren't finding some transcendental state of calm where the mind goes blank. Quite the contrary, mindfulness meditation is not about clearing our mind; it's about *observing* our mind in all its glorious activity. It's the nature of the mind to be active and busy. I would be worried if someone observed a blank mind—they might be dead!

I explained this to Mia and urged her to try it again. "Mindfulness is experiential. Take a leap of faith with me and give it a try while you are doing this program. I promise, if you still hate it when our time is up, you never have to meditate again."

Mia agreed and, along with the other group participants, she developed a daily mindfulness practice. At the beginning it was tough, but while she didn't exactly look forward to the practice, it was only five minutes a day and she stuck with it. Over time it became part of her routine, and it felt weird on the days that she didn't meditate, kind of like she had forgotten to brush her teeth. She started to notice what her mind and body were telling her, initially observing the activities of her mind and body during the five-minute meditation and then expanding this awareness outside of the meditation practice as well. She noticed that she was hungry earlier in the day and started to eat breakfast. She felt better when she ate regularly throughout the day in accordance to her hunger signals, stopping when she felt satisfied, and choosing foods that she enjoyed and made her body feel good. She started to feel less out of control around food, and while she still enjoyed eating from her favorite restaurants, she no longer berated herself afterward. She still ordered multiple dishes if she wanted them all, but now she usually had leftovers, which she would enjoy for a meal the next day. You'll learn more about eating in tune to hunger, fullness and satiation, taste, and mindful choices in chapters 5–8, but it all starts with mindfulness.

What Is Mindfulness?

Have you ever seen a sunset so beautiful that it felt as if you were taking in the dazzling array of colors with every cell in your body? Or had the experience of gazing into the eyes of a newborn baby and been so enraptured that it was as if nothing else in the world mattered? Perhaps you have played (or watched) a sport where your attention was razor-focused on where the ball was at any given millisecond in time? Or been so completely captivated by a piece of music that your full self was swept up with the sound? Have you ever suffered a migraine headache so intense that all you could do is feel every painful sensation in your body? Or had such great sex that you lost sense of time and all that you perceived was the pleasure you were experiencing in that moment?

All of these are examples of mindfulness, the experience of being fully present in the current moment. Mindfulness has been cultivated through meditative practices in religious traditions for thousands of years. While mindfulness is most commonly associated with Buddhism, it has roots in many different religions including Hinduism, Judaism, Christianity, and Islam. In the 1970s Jon Kabat-Zinn, a scientist and longtime meditator in the Zen Buddhist tradition, brought mindfulness practices into Western medical settings. He secularized the practice and created the Mindfulness-Based Stress Reduction (MBSR) program, a research-based eight-week program initially developed to help people struggling with chronic pain. In an interview about the development of MBSR, Kabat-Zinn recalls a conversation he had with physicians at University of Massachusetts Medical Center in which they estimated that only 20 percent of patients were being helped by the traditional medical treatments available.[1] The other 80 percent of patients were simply falling through the cracks. Kabat-Zinn believed that meditation could be a powerful tool to help these people—and he was right.

Today hundreds of published research studies support the benefits of mindfulness. The strongest evidence supports the effectiveness of mindfulness in the treatment of chronic pain, depression, and anxiety, but there are also studies suggesting that mindfulness can be helpful in reducing high blood pressure, psoriasis, fibromyalgia, and post-traumatic stress disorder and improving immune response, brain functioning, sleep, and overall health. It's ubiquitous in self-help, productivity, and performance settings, with applications to parenting, relationships, sports, and work. A number of *Fortune* 500 companies have integrated mindfulness into employee wellness, and Google even has a chief mindfulness officer on staff. While this book will focus on the application of mindfulness to eating and body image, it relies on many of the same meditation practices used in all of the other types of mindfulness-based treatments—so don't be surprised if you start to see changes in other areas of your life as well.

Research suggests that mindfulness is effective in the treatment of eating disorders and disordered eating, especially binge-eating disorder. A 2020 review study that analyzed nine published randomized controlled trials (considered the "gold standard" in research methodology) concluded that mindfulness and/or mindful eating were associated with reduced binge eating, decreased emotional eating, less eating in response to external cues, fewer weight and shape concerns, increased self-acceptance, and better regulation of emotions.[2] Another review that analyzed the results of twenty-four peer-reviewed studies found that when we eat mindlessly, our brain—specifically the parts of our brain related to memory—doesn't register the full extent of the meal.[3] When we eat without being fully present (as we do when we are in conflict with food), we tend to eat more not only during the meal but also later on. This is because we underestimate how much we ate and compensate for it at the next meal. In addition, when we aren't paying attention we don't enjoy our food as much, leaving us feeling unsatisfied and wanting more.

When we aren't eating in accordance with our "internal GPS," discussed later in this chapter, we rely on our memory to make decisions around food. When our memories are impaired or were never fully encoded because we weren't present for the eating experience, this guidance becomes less reliable. Mindfulness helps us tune in to our internal GPS, a more reliable system to guide our eating.

Mindful eating is simply about becoming aware of what your body needs in any given moment and using that information to make informed decisions about how to move forward with your own best interests in mind. The goal of mindful eating, as taught in this book, is not to eat less food. While it is an understandable inclination to bring diet mentality into mindful eating (after all, these old thoughts, feelings, and influences are deeply ingrained and aren't just going to disappear overnight), if you make mindful eating about eating less or eating only "healthy" foods, you've just turned it into a diet plan. (And remember, diets don't work.) Instead, the intention is to let your body guide your eating. Sometimes you will be surprised at how much food your body is calling for, and sometimes you will be shocked that you don't want something you never could've imagined leaving behind—both of these are a good thing! We must celebrate both of these accomplishments with the same vigor. The time that we leave half a slice of cake behind on our plate is just as amazing as the time you enjoy two slices.

There is a reason that mindfulness practices have been applied so widely: they not only treat specific symptoms, but they also fundamentally change how you relate to yourself and the world around you. Studies suggest that mindfulness meditation even changes the wiring in your brain! One study, published in 2011, conducted MRI brain scans before and after participants went through an eight-week MBSR program.[4] These people had never meditated prior to starting the program. Following the meditation program, scans revealed an increase in gray matter density in the brain, specifically in brain regions associated with learning and memory processes, emotion regulation, self-referential processing, and perspective taking. A 2014 paper that reviewed more than twenty different research studies concluded that mindfulness is associated with changes in eight regions of the brain, including areas associated with self-regulation, learning from past experiences, emotion, memory, and stress.[5] Other studies have found changes in the brain regions associated with perception, body awareness, pain tolerance, emotion regulation, introspection, complex thinking, and sense of self.[6] It is important to note that these changes are observed in novice meditators—people, perhaps like you, who are just starting to practice meditation for the first time—and these changes are observed over a relatively short period of time (often two months) with meditation practice periods of less than thirty minutes.

Jon Kabat-Zinn defines mindfulness as "awareness that arises through paying attention, on purpose, in the present moment, nonjudgmentally."[7] Mindfulness naturally occurs at certain moments in life, often when we are doing things that captivate and fully engage us, and it is also a state that we can cultivate through meditation and practices, as we will do in this book. Mindfulness is inherently experiential. In his book *Full Catastrophe Living*, Kabat-Zinn explains that "cultivating mindfulness is not unlike the process of eating. It would be absurd to propose that someone else eat for you. And when you go to a restaurant, you don't eat the menu, mistaking it for the meal, nor are you nourished by listening to the waiter describe the food. You have to actually eat the food for it to nourish you. In the same way, you have to actually practice mindfulness, by which I mean cultivate it systematically in your own life, in order to reap its benefits and come to understand why it is so valuable."[8] I've told you about the research studies finding mindfulness useful in improving disordered eating and body image, and I'll do my best to explain mindfulness to you, but it is only through your own regular meditation practice that you will truly understand what it means to be mindful.

Your Internal GPS

Did you know that your body comes hardwired with a powerful system to guide your eating? Believe it or not, we were able to figure out what, when, and how much to eat long before dieting was invented! In fact, since our earliest days as humans, our survival has depended on our ability to eat in ways that nourish our body and keep us alive.

Your appetite regulation system, or what I call your "internal GPS," is the guidance system that helps you decide what, when, and how much to eat. It includes cues like hunger, fullness, satiation, taste of foods, cravings, preferences for different foods and styles of eating, and how your body reacts to certain foods. If you are driving in your car and don't know your route, without your GPS turned on it's impossible to know which way to go. The same is true of our internal GPS to guide our eating—without it, we are lost.

Over the years, most of us have become disconnected from our body's internal GPS. We may even believe that we don't have one or that ours is broken. This is what we've been taught, that we cannot trust our own body. In all but the most unusual of circumstances, you *do* have an internal GPS system and it is *not* broken. If you think that you fall into that bucket of "the most unusual of circumstances," I'll tell you now that you probably don't. We always think we are the exception to the rule. Of course, if you think that you have a medical problem that is affecting your appetite, a consult with your medical doctor is a good idea. If you are struggling with an eating disorder, consulting with your treatment provider is essential. For most of us, though, the volume of our GPS is just turned down low, so we need a little practice in learning how to hear it. Interference from diet culture also makes it difficult to hear our internal GPS. Imagine you are driving in your car with the volume of the navigation system turned all the way down *and* you are blasting loud music from amped-up speakers. Is it any surprise that you can't hear the quiet voice of your navigation?

Mindfulness is the key to turning up the volume on your internal GPS. That's why developing a regular meditation practice is a central part of this program—it's the instrument that allows you to hear the wisdom of your body. Diet culture is like the music blasting over the quiet navigation system; it is the interference that makes it hard to hear the directions your internal GPS is giving you. That's why the first two chapters in this book were dedicated to leaving diet culture behind. It is impossible to honor your internal cues when you are in conflict with your body, when you mistrust your body, and when you are overriding the signals your body is sending you.

As you move away from a reliance on external cues, like dieting, to guide your eating, you'll be tuning in to your body's wealth of internal wisdom, your internal GPS. This is a more reliable, sustainable, and peaceful way of eating that works with what your body naturally wants to do instead of trying to fight against your body. (And as we learned in chapter 1, fighting against your body is almost always a losing battle. Besides, you have so many more important things to do in life than be at war with yourself!) Your internal cues—hunger, satiation, taste, cravings, preferences, and more—are customized uniquely for you because they come from your own body. It may not feel like your body is sending you wisdom right now, but I promise you it's there. We'll do a deep dive into each of these components of our internal GPS in chapters 5–8.

In contrast to our internal GPS, external cues are unreliable and not attuned to your body's unique needs. External cues include things like how much food is on your plate, what time of day it is (e.g., it's noon and that means it is time to eat lunch, or it's 10 p.m. and that is too late to eat even though I feel hungry), when, what, and how much food you are served, and what the "experts" tell us to eat. They are one-size-fits-all cues that often have absolutely nothing to do with what is best for our bodies. Dieting is focused on ignoring our internal cues to prioritize guidance from outside sources. In this book you're learning to shift your focus to your internal cues and embrace the wisdom of the person who knows how to care for you the best—you!

Many advice columns simplify mindful eating to just eating distraction-free. Turn off the television, close your computer, step away from your phone, and—poof—we are magically good to go. But if it were that easy you wouldn't have bought this book. It's hard to sit down, just you and your food. It's hard to listen to your body. It's hard to be present with yourself. One of the reasons mindful eating is so challenging is because diet culture makes us doubt the integrity of our internal signals. It creates turmoil around food and painful emotional reactions that we want to run away from. Distracted eating is appealing; when our eating experiences are filled with conflict and distress, it is more comfortable to tune out with television or a podcast or to eat quickly without much thought. But while distraction and avoidance may have appeal, ignorance is not bliss. It is impossible to change things that we are not aware of. When we are tuned out, we are likely to repeat the same cycles again and again, even if those cycles make us miserable.

Increasing our awareness through mindfulness meditation is the first step to changing unwanted patterns and behaviors in our life. Mindfulness helps us become more aware of our thoughts, feelings, and behaviors in any given moment while cultivating a sense of nonjudgmental acceptance. Without mindful awareness, we are like passengers in an out-of-control car being taken on a wild ride. Awareness helps us get back in the driver's seat, make conscious decisions, and regain a sense of control. Hopefully, based on what you've learned in chapters 1 and 2, this conflict is starting to lessen (even just a tiny bit) as we realize that your body was never the problem. The problem is diet culture. Increasing our self-compassion and self-acceptance, as we'll be learning to do in the next chapter, will also help reduce the conflict within ourselves and free up the path to sitting with our own body and being present for our eating experiences.

Establishing a Mindfulness Practice

Neuroplasticity is the brain's ability to change over time in response to our experiences. Mindfulness practice is associated with changes in the brain, specifically in the areas of self-awareness, emotion regulation, compassion, and stress. Think of meditation as strength training for your brain. Imagine doing bicep curls with weights. The first time you do the movement, it may feel unfamiliar and uncomfortable. You may worry that you are doing it wrong. You may not see any noticeable changes in your strength after any single training session. You may check out your muscles in the mirror and notice that they look the same. *Is this really working? Is there any point to continuing?* But if you develop a consistent routine, over time the exercises may start to feel more natural. You may be able to lift more weight and notice muscle definition. Most importantly, when someone hands you a heavy package or you are called upon to open that unforgiving jar of pickles in the kitchen, that muscle is there for you when you need it. Your own strength may even surprise you. A consistent meditation practice is what builds up the muscle in your brain (or rewires the neurological pathways, to be more specific) to allow you to call on the skills you are learning in this book, in the moments that you need them most.

Meditation needs to be accessible. Rather than creating a space to meditate that we go *out* to, we want to create a space within our everyday life that we can easily come *in* to. You want to build a meditation practice that works in your life, tailored to your unique needs. We are going to start with the intention of meditating for five minutes each day. All you need is a device to listen to the guided meditation and a place to meditate. We are going to start off practicing with a guided meditation, but once you've gotten the hang of things, you can also just set a timer for five minutes and lead yourself through the practice if you prefer.

When you think about meditation, you may imagine someone sitting in full lotus position, cross-legged on the floor with each foot on the opposite thigh, looking all Zen. You may picture a special place designed for meditation—an ashram, a monastery, or a meditation center. Or you may think about special equipment like a meditation cushion, a meditation chime or singing bowl, some candles, or even a little altar. While these things can be pretty and nice, none is required for meditation. In the words of Winston Churchill, "Perfection is the enemy of progress." It doesn't make sense to build an altar or spend money on fancy cushions if you never use them. The ideal silent location isn't so ideal if you aren't there when it's time to meditate. Here in New York City, the subway can be a great place to meditate. It is far from silent, you are surrounded by people, and you may not even be able to get a seat; but it is a well-integrated part of our daily routine and we are a captive audience, so it's hard to find an excuse for why we can't pop in our earbuds and listen to a five-minute guided meditation. For people who live with young kids or large families, the bathroom can become a meditation sanctuary. It's often one of the few doors with a lock on it, if you are lucky people will leave you alone for five minutes, plus as a bonus it already has a (toilet) seat! A parked car can become a sacred place if you sit for a five-minute meditation before transitioning to the next place you are going. There is no right or wrong when it comes to meditation. The best way to meditate is the way that you meditate—whether that is sitting on a cushion in a special meditation room that you've designed or sitting on the toilet in your bathroom. Both are equally awesome. Don't get lost in searching for perfection; just do what you think will work best for you and see how it goes. If it turns out that place doesn't work, try somewhere else. This is a process of flexible experimentation.

Ideally, if it is available to you, choose a place that is quiet, where you won't be interrupted, and where you can sit down. I recommend sitting in a straight-backed chair (like a dining chair) where your hips are positioned higher than your knees. If you want, you can experiment with sitting on a meditation cushion (also called a *zafu*), perhaps with a flatter cushion (a *zabuton*) or a blanket underneath to protect your knees and ankles from the hard floor. Keep in mind that there are no special benefits to sitting on the floor to meditate. Sitting in a chair has the same effect, and many people find this to be more comfortable (especially when it's time to get up!). When you take your seat to meditate, try to sit with a straight upright posture, using your core to hold you up without leaning against the backrest of the chair. Try to find a position where your spine is naturally aligned; it can be useful to rock back and forth a bit in your seat to find this position. As always, be flexible. If this position isn't comfortable or accessible to you, take whatever position your body is calling for. If you have medical issues that make it uncomfortable to sit, try standing up or lying down.

Building a meditation practice is building a habit. Habits thrive on consistency. Identify a consistent time and place to meditate each day. It doesn't matter when and where you choose, but make it part of your daily schedule. If we don't have a game plan each day for when and where we will meditate, it is easy to push it off. *Now isn't a good time, I'll meditate later.* Before you know it, it's time to go to bed and you never meditated. Avoid aspirational meditation goals. For example, if you are someone who struggles to get out of bed in the morning, hitting snooze over and over until you are running late and rushing out the door, don't use this as your moment to become someone who wakes up and meditates at 5 a.m. Similarly, if you are not someone who regularly goes to the gym, don't intend to mediate each day after you go to the gym. Don't make it more difficult by designing a practice for the person you want to be; create a routine that will work best for the person you actually are.

Do you have any routines that you do every day? Could you add the five-minute meditation into that routine? For example, if you always take a shower, get dressed, then brush your teeth, might you be able to shower, get dressed, meditate, and then brush your teeth? Research suggests that attaching a new behavior to existing habits creates a chain of events that we easily move through in sequence.[9] Over time that new behavior (meditation in this case) becomes a habit. If you don't have any daily routines that you can add meditation to, choose a consistent time of day, 9 a.m. or noon for example, and set an alarm to remind you to meditate each day at that time no matter what you are doing.

While finding a consistent time and place to meditate is ideal, flexibility is important too. If the time and place that you initially choose wind up not working for you, by all means change it up. If you don't think you can meditate at the same time and place each day, try a few different times and places. This is a process of experimenting to discover what works best for you.

Habits aren't formed overnight. One study suggests that it takes an average of sixty-six days, or a little over two months, to build a habit.[10] But the amount of time it takes for a behavior to become a habit can vary quite a bit from person to person, so try to be patient, trust in the process, and stick with it. If you miss a day—or even miss a week or more—no big deal; when you feel ready, come back to your practice with a sense of compassion and gentleness.

Do you keep falling asleep when you meditate? This is a common hazard of meditation. Many of us are so chronically sleep deprived that as soon as we close our eyes to meditate, our bodies go right into sleep mode. And that is okay. If you feel exhausted, listen to your body and allow yourself to sleep. The intention of meditation is not to fall asleep but rather, in the words of Jon Kabat-Zinn, to fall awake.[11] If you end up snoozing through your meditation time, come back to the meditation practice at another time. If you are consistently falling asleep when you meditate, try meditating at a different time of day. Many people find that if they meditate in the evening, especially right before bed, they are prone to falling asleep. See if you stay more alert if you meditate in the morning or afternoon. You can also try standing up to meditate or keeping your eyes open during the practice. It's also important to make sure that you are getting enough rest, as we'll discuss in chapter 10.

Breathing Mindful Breaths

We will build our meditation habit using a "mindfulness of breath" practice. Let's try this practice now. Take a seat in the meditative position described earlier, with your feet flat on the ground and your spine upright, or whatever position your body is calling for. Either close your eyes gently or keep them open with a soft unfocused gaze down toward the ground in front of you. Bring your full awareness to your breath, noticing the breath as it enters and exits your body. There is no need to change your breath in any way; simply observe what your body is already doing. Just notice the breath as it enters and exits your body. You may find that your attention is called to some aspect of the breath, perhaps the sound that the breath makes as it enters and exits through your nostrils or passes through your throat, the rhythmic expansion of your belly as it fills with air and contraction as it releases the air back out to the world, or the temperature of the air, cooler as it enters your body and warmer as it exits. Whatever it is, allow your attention to rest fully with your breath.

Over time you will likely notice your mind wandering away from the breath. This is natural and to be expected. When you have noticed that your mind has wandered off, simply observe this and, without judgment, gently bring your attention back to the breath. Repeat this process of focusing your full awareness on breath, noticing when your mind has wandered off, and compassionately bringing your awareness back to your breath for the duration of the meditation. You can either set a timer for five minutes and walk yourself through this process or go to www.drconason.com /diet-free-revolution/ and listen to the five-minute guided exercise on mindfulness of breath.

When practicing mindfulness of breath, it is easy to get misled and believe that the point of the meditation is to stay completely focused on your breath for the entire meditation period. If your mind wanders away from the breath and you become distracted, you may believe that you are doing the meditation wrong. You're not! It's the nature of the mind to be busy, to become distracted, to wander away from the breath. It is the moments when we notice that our mind has wandered off that are true mindfulness. The breath is a tool to observe the activity of the mind. The intention of the practice is not to observe the breath but rather to observe the mind.

Think of the breath as an anchor point that we keep coming back to during the practice, similar to how a boat is anchored in rough waters. The boat won't stay completely centered on the anchor—it will drift a bit here and there—but the anchor will keep the boat from going too far astray and getting lost at sea. During a meditation practice, your mind will wander off. Simply notice when your mind has wandered off and gently refocus your awareness on your breathing. It is this process of using the breath as an anchor—observing your mind straying from your breath and gently bringing your mind back to focus on your breath—that is the mindfulness practice. In fact, each moment that our mind wanders off and we notice this and are able to refocus our awareness back on our breath is a true moment of mindfulness. A busy mind doesn't mean that you are a bad meditator or that you are meditating wrong; it just means that you have plenty of opportunities to mindfully observe your beautifully busy mind in action.

Taking a Mindful Pause

We will also use a short meditative practice that I call a "mindful pause." This is a brief meditative moment that allows us to become fully present in the here and now. You can find a guided mindful pause meditation at www.drconason.com/diet-free-revolution/. During a mindful pause, we follow these five steps:

1. Bring your full awareness to your breath for two to five breath cycles.

2. Expand your awareness to focus on your body.

3. Notice if there is anything that your body is trying to communicate to you. Do you feel hunger, fullness, satiation, cravings, aches or pains, sensations of pleasure or discomfort, or anything else?

4. Notice if there is anything that your mind is trying to communicate to you. Are there any emotions arising at this moment? Do you feel happy, sad, stressed, hurt, anxious, bored, angry, or anything else?

5. How can you best tend to any needs you notice? What do you need in this moment, and how can you best care for yourself? How can you move forward with kindness and compassion?

As you learn about the different aspects of your internal GPS in the following chapters, you will use the mindful pause as a way to tune in to each component, including hunger, fullness, taste, cravings and desires, your body's reactions to foods, and more. The mindful pause can be used before, during, and after eating to become fully present with your body and eating experiences. In addition to helping you tune in to your internal GPS, you can also use the mindful pause to check in with yourself throughout the day. Think about how often you ask other people how they are doing. How often do you ask yourself the same question? The mindful pause is an opportunity to assess how you are doing at any moment in time and see if there is anything you need. You can use this meditative moment to become aware of any thoughts, feelings, and bodily sensations that need tending to throughout the day.

You may be familiar with a mindful moment before eating that is found in many different religious traditions. In Christianity it is a common practice to "say grace" before a meal. In Judaism there is a hand-washing ritual, and prayers are said for different foods. In Islam prayers are said before eating to bless the meal. In fact, in almost all religions examples can be found for a sacred pause before eating and a moment of gratitude for the food and all involved in bringing that food to the table. While they may not call it mindfulness, in essence it is taking a moment of reflection to recognize that eating is a sacred activity apart from the typical hustle and bustle of the rest of the day. Whether you call it grace, prayer, or a mindful pause, the importance of taking a moment to pause, reflect, and express gratitude is an ancient tradition that helps us prepare for the eating experience. We don't have to be religious to enjoy the benefits that this mindful pause can bring.

Can I just skip the meditation part? I get it. Sitting with ourselves is hard. Meditation can feel boring. Uncomfortable feelings may arise. There are other things that you want to do with that five minutes of your life. I wish I knew a way to give you the benefits of mindfulness without practicing meditation. But we really do need to practice meditation to get the benefits. I truly believe that it is the most powerful tool we have to radically transform our relationship with food, our body, and ourselves. Mindfulness practice is the foundation for everything else in this book. It will help increase your awareness of your body's internal sensations and develop your observational capacities so that you can hear, honor, and nourish your body's innate needs. Mindfulness also fosters our ability to notice our thoughts and emotions so that we can make conscious informed choices about how we want to act, rather than reacting or being stuck in autopilot mode. Through these skills, along with the acceptance and compassion (which you'll learn about in the next chapter) inherent in mindfulness, you can work toward being less conflicted and can free yourself to be more present in your relationship with food, your body, and the world around you.

TAKE-ACTION ACTIVITIES

Meditate daily with five minutes of mindful breath

Go to www.drconason.com/diet-free-revolution/ to listen to the guided meditation that I have recorded for you. Most people find it useful to listen to a guided meditation when learning to meditate. Once you've gotten the feel for meditating using the guided meditation, you can experiment with setting a timer for five minutes and guiding yourself through the meditation practice. Play with what works best for you, the guided meditation or the timer, equally good options. You will continue with this daily mindfulness meditation practice for the duration of this program, and perhaps even beyond that!

Identify a time and place where you plan to meditate. Experiment and see how this time and place work for you. If it doesn't work, be flexible and try something else. Remember: the best time and place to meditate is the time and place that you meditate. Done is better than perfect.

If possible, integrate your daily meditation practice into a daily routine that you already effortlessly engage in. This could be your morning hygiene routine, what you do when you first arrive at work, or your evening care ritual.

Set your intention! Schedule your meditation time in your calendar, and protect that time from being infringed upon by other activities.

Integrate the mindful pause into your daily routine

Set an alert or reminder on your phone or other device to go off at random intervals as a reminder to take mindful pauses throughout the day. Countless apps have this function, including mindfulness ones that mimic the sounds of chimes, bells, or gongs. You can also have the alarm on your phone go off at set times during the day, which even the most basic phone models usually come with. Whenever this alert goes off, take a few seconds to check in with yourself. Ask yourself: *How am I doing right now? Is there anything I need?* If you are in the middle of doing something, don't hit snooze! Just pause for a few seconds and see how you are doing. Even if you are in a meeting or in the middle of an activity, you can become fully present with yourself without anyone else even realizing. Whatever you are doing will still be there a few seconds later.

Prior to eating, take a mindful pause to check in with your body and become present with your food. Do you notice any bodily sensations of hunger or fullness? Any cravings? We are going to learn about hunger, fullness, and cravings later in this book, so don't worry if you have a tough time deciphering these signals right now. Use your senses to take in as much as you can about the appearance, smell, textures, and tastes of the food. Is the food appetizing? Do you like it?

Apply your mindfulness skills to your eating

Just as you've practiced becoming fully present with your breath, you can practice becoming fully present with your food. Choose something to eat. This basic mindful eating exercise is most commonly done with raisins, but feel free to choose another item if you prefer, perhaps a piece of fruit, some cheese, or a cookie. If there is any wrapping or packaging, take the food out now. Start out by examining the food item. Notice as much as you can about the food with your eyes. What color is it? What shape is it? Is it uniform or do parts of the food look different? Is there a sheen or texture? You can also use your fingers to explore the food. What does it feel like? Is it squishy, tough, rough, soft, or smooth? Bring the item up to your nose and smell it. What do you notice about the scent?

Once you have explored the object using your eyes, hands, and nose, bring a piece of the food up to your mouth. Press the item against the outside of your lips and notice if any sensations arise. What textures do your lips detect? Do you notice any sensations happening in your mouth as you prepare to eat the food? Perhaps salivation? When you are ready, place the food in your mouth and hold it there without biting into it. Do you notice any taste? Textures or sensations in your mouth? Bite into the food and start chewing slowly. Does the taste change at all? Notice as much as you can as you eat this item, swallowing the bite of food when ready. Do any sensations linger in your mouth or body after you have swallowed the bite?

When you have finished eating this morsel of food, take another piece of the food and lead yourself through the process of examining it with your eyes and hands, bringing it to your nose and smelling it, holding it for a moment to the outside of your lips, and then placing it in your mouth and noting the taste of the food as you chew and eventually swallow, noticing if any sensations remain after you swallow. Then take a third piece of the food. Again lead yourself through the process of examining it with your eyes and fingers and bring it up to your nose and smell it. Do you want to eat this bite? If so, walk yourself through mindfully eating the third bite of food, placing it in your mouth and noticing as much as you can about the taste of this food. Continue to eat in this manner, using all your senses to take in as much as you can about the eating experience, until you feel satisfied and no longer want to continue eating. (A guided audio version of this meditation using a raisin is available at www.drconason.com/diet-free-revolution/.)

This exercise is a practice designed to build mindful eating skills. It's not practical to eat in this way all the time. Mindful eating can be practiced while eating quickly, on the go, even in front of the television. It's simply about bringing our full awareness to our eating. What elements of this exercise can you bring to other eating experiences this week? Journal about your experiences with mindful eating—write down what you noticed, felt, thought, tasted, or whatever comes to mind.

4

STEP 4: You Are Not Broken
How to Become a Kind Companion to Yourself

*T*racy had hated her body for as long as she could remember. While she had always been taught that her body was bad, an experience at her pediatrician's office when she was ten years old stands out in her mind. Sitting on the exam table at the doctor's office, she felt the thin white paper crinkle under her bottom, which, in a moment, she would be told was unacceptably large. Her pediatrician loomed over her. He was a tall, thin man, skeletal almost, his pointy nose holding up narrow wire-frame glasses that he peered over as he looked alternately at Tracy, at the file that he held in front of him, then back at Tracy. "What are we going to do about this?" Now he looked accusingly at Tracy's mother, who sat on a stool beside her. "She's far too big." He shook his head as he held out a piece of paper with a chart and a mark at the upper-right-hand corner. "Ninety-second percentile. That's no place for a young lady to be. You'll have to do something." The corners of his mouth turned downward in an expression that could only be interpreted as disgust.

Tracy tugged her shoulders inward, willing herself to become smaller as her face flushed red. She studied the beige-and-white speckled tiles on the floor, wishing that the earth would open up and whisk her away from the growing sense of shame. She was embarrassed not only for herself but also for her mother, whose face had turned an even deeper shade of crimson.

Even at her young age, Tracy knew that her mother's body—the one that looked so similar to her own—was bad and shameful. Tracy and her mother drove home in silence. Tracy knew that her mom wasn't angry with her; it was something far worse. Her own body had revealed her mother's body—what her mother had spent a lifetime trying to hide was suddenly laid bare in the doctor's judgment. She had become the cause of her mother's shame, a shame that ran so deep it was unspeakable.

Earlier that day, when Tracy's mother had reminded her that they had the pediatrician appointment after school, Tracy had asked if they could stop at the Dairy Queen on their way back home. Her mother had agreed to the special treat, and Tracy had been looking forward to getting an ice cream sundae and enjoying some special time, just the two of them. As they drove home, the neon DQ sign loomed in the distance. As they got closer and closer, neither Tracy nor her mother spoke a word. The car didn't slow for even a moment. As quickly as the sign had appeared, it shrank in the rearview mirror until it was completely out of sight. Tracy knew there would be no more ice cream in her future.

Once home Tracy went straight to her room, got out her pink journal with an image of a ballerina on the cover, unlocked it with the tiny key she kept in her nightstand, and started writing her most private thoughts. *I want to lose weight. I want to lose weight. I want to lose weight.* She wrote the phrase over and over until her fingers cramped up and her eyes were so blurry with tears she could hardly see. She vowed to forsake all sweets, carbs, fats, and any other foods that would come between her and this goal.

It's been more than thirty years but tears still sting at her eyes when she thinks back to it. Over the years, the shame surrounding her body has only grown as her body continued to expand. While she no longer writes in her pink journal, Tracy's deepest wish remained the same as when she was ten: lose weight. But despite everything she has tried to do to tame her body into submission, it had remained uncooperative. Like so many women, Tracy developed a cruel inner voice that taunted her day and night. *You're disgusting. Look at you shoving food into your face, you have no self-control. It's no wonder your husband hardly looks at you anymore. Who would want to sleep with a cow?* This voice was relentless. But despite her belief that cruelty would motivate her to get her eating in check, the incessant self-flagellation only seemed to fuel her nightly binge-eating episodes.

Basic psychology teaches us that punishment is not an effective motivator for behavior change. If you ever took an Intro to Psych class, you probably learned about famed behaviorist B. F. Skinner. In the 1940s he did a series of experiments that involved putting a rat in a box and giving it electric shocks as punishment for certain behaviors. Sounds like a fun guy, right? Regardless of how he liked to get his kicks, his experiments taught us something important about punishment—it doesn't work. Rather than decrease unwanted behaviors, punishment caused generalized fear and aggression, Skinner found.[1] After being exposed to punishment, the rats basically cowered in the corner of the cage and tried to bite whoever tried to stick their hand in to feed them.

In the 1960s psychologist Martin Seligman built on Skinner's work. While the punishment that Skinner's rats endured was linked to behaviors that the rats could change, Seligman created a condition where electric shocks were given at random to dogs that had no ability to stop the shocks. The dogs developed what he termed "learned helplessness."[2] When the dogs were later given the ability to stop the shocks, they made no efforts to change their environment—they just lay there being shocked, having apparently given up hope that they could ever make it stop. Each time we berate ourselves, we are like that animal in Skinner's (or even worse, Seligman's) box giving ourselves an electric shock. Berating ourselves is not going to change our behavior—it just terrorizes us.

But if I am kinder to myself, I'll never change my behavior. This is a concern many of my clients have when we talk about quieting our inner critic. And I totally understand that concern; after all, diet culture teaches us "no pain, no gain." But if berating yourself was effective, you wouldn't be here right now reading this book. Rather than being the vehicle for change, negative self-talk is associated with decreased motivation, increased feelings of helplessness, increased stress, and increased risk of mental health problems, research suggests.[3] Internalized weight bias, which rears its head in our cruel inner dialogue, is associated with (among other things) increased eating disorders and disordered eating, loss of control eating, emotional eating, and body image dissatisfaction.[4] Rather than criticism and punishment, it is acceptance and compassion that set the stage for change.

Intuitively this makes a lot of sense. We know that, for example, if we are cruel to a child, the most likely outcome is that the child becomes terrorized, traumatized, and filled with shame; seldom is abuse the path toward making children happy or successful. The most well-adjusted children are those with kind and loving parents who nurture and strive to hold the child's best interests in mind. These parents encourage the child to be their authentic self, not who the parents want them to be. These same principles hold true for us. As adults, we need to treat ourselves with the same love and respect with which a good parent would treat a child. Despite the obvious detrimental effects of abuse in others, many of us continue to believe that berating ourselves will lead to weight loss. It's like we think, *If I just hate myself enough, if I can just make myself miserable enough, surely I'll find the motivation to make changes in my life.* If self-criticism led to weight loss, we would be a nation underweight. Rather than being the impetus for change, our harsh inner critic keeps us immobilized.

We are our own worst critics. And for good reason! As we've been learning, there is a lot invested in us believing that we are flawed. Diet culture, which we know to be an amalgam of oppressive racist, Eurocentric, patriarchal beauty norms, creates a fertile ground for shame, defined as the belief that you are bad. Unlike guilt or embarrassment, where negative feelings are directed toward your *behavior* (i.e., I *did* something bad and I feel guilty or embarrassed), with shame the negative feelings are directed toward *you* (i.e., I *am* bad). Philosopher Hilge Landweer theorizes that shame occurs when a person has transgressed a norm viewed as desirable and binding.[5] Diet culture, and the systems of oppression that support it, creates social norms that we can't help but transgress. How many of us look like the impossibly thin, prepubescent, white, femme ideals that diet culture puts forth? How many of us can consistently perform the restrictive, anhedonic, self-sacrificing norms that diet culture demands? Is it any wonder that most of us grapple with deep feelings of shame? How can we ever feel good enough when we are told practically from birth that we are flawed and our value stems from achieving unattainable ideals?

Our harsh inner critic is an internalization of these demands. *Be thinner, have more self-control, your body is unacceptable, you are unlovable, it is all your fault.* We are convinced that we need to be harsh toward ourselves because we cannot be trusted with kindness. If we were gentler with ourselves, we are afraid we would "let ourselves go." Self-acceptance is seen as a sign of defeat; we believe that if we accept ourselves as we are, we'll lose any motivation to change.

Understandably it is terrifying to imagine being stuck in that place of self-hatred forever. We all just want to escape the misery of self-loathing, and we are taught that changing our body is the path out. But there is another way. Self-compassion and acceptance, two essential components of mindfulness, are the antidotes to shame and self-hatred.

Self-compassion is the process of approaching yourself with a fundamental stance of kindness and finding ways to care for and comfort yourself in times of difficulty and suffering. Psychologist and self-compassion expert Kristin Neff defines self-compassion as involving three components: self-kindness (being warm toward yourself in the face of pain or personal shortcomings), common humanity (recognizing that suffering and personal failures are part of the shared human experience), and mindfulness (observing emotions with nonjudgmental detached open awareness).[6] Self-compassion is associated with a bunch of positive outcomes including increased happiness, optimism, positive affect, curiosity and exploration, productivity, and decreased stress.[7] It's been shown to enhance psychological well-being, enable warm relationships with others, and increase self-acceptance.[8] In a study examining the effect of self-compassion on body image, researchers found that practicing a daily twenty-minute self-compassion meditation for three weeks was associated with decreased body dissatisfaction, body shame, and contingent self-worth based on appearance (i.e., valuing yourself based on what you look like); participants increased their self-compassion and body appreciation.[9]

Imagine that you encounter a child who is crying. For most of us, our instinct is to try and comfort the child, lovingly ask what is wrong, perhaps put a caring arm around them or reassure the child that they are loved and cared for. Our heart may even ache a bit to see a child cry as we identify with the child's pain and feel their sadness with them. This is compassion. The word *compassion* comes from the Latin for "suffer with" and has been described by Neff as our heart responding to another's pain. While compassion may be our natural inclination when we see a child suffering, our reaction to our own hurt is quite different. Think about a time when you ate in a way that felt problematic. How did you respond to yourself? Did you offer yourself kindness and compassion? Did you say to yourself, *Wow, that was rough, You're struggling right now, poor thing, what can we do to help you, what do you need in this moment?* If you are anything like me in my dieting days, this was probably not your first response. My inner dialogue was more along the lines of *what the hell is wrong with you, you are such a loser, why did you eat like that again?* We say things to ourselves that we wouldn't say to our worst enemies. Rather than supporting ourselves with love and compassion, we kick ourselves when we are down. It's like falling down one step, scraping our knee, and then instead of getting an ice pack and bandage, we shove ourselves down the remaining flight of steps. And then when we are injured at the bottom of the stairs, we blame ourselves for having difficulty getting back up. Hopefully we can all agree that this strategy is not working out so well.

How can I offer myself compassion when I don't like myself? I'm often asked this by my clients. It can be hard to imagine offering yourself kindness when you are immersed in self-hatred. Imagine the small child from our earlier example (or feel free to sub in a cute puppy here if that's more your speed). For anyone who has ever spent time around kids (or puppies), you know that they don't always behave the way that you want them to. Sometimes they drive us completely up the wall. Maybe your kid is whining because you won't let them watch more television. Or perhaps your puppy peed all over your brand-new rug. Can you call to mind a time that a child or puppy or someone you love unconditionally did something that you didn't like? Do you remember what you felt in that moment? You probably felt angry. But you also may have been able to hold on to a sense of love for the child or puppy and fundamentally want the best for them, even in the moment of anger. Even at the maddest I've been with my kids, I may hate their behavior and fantasize about running away to a Caribbean island to live out the rest of my days alone with an endless supply of piña coladas (or is that just me?), but I still love them. Even when I'm angry, even in a moment of hatred, I don't want to really hurt them. And if in the middle of a blowout argument, my daughter tripped and fell, my heart would ache for her and I would run to make sure that she was okay. If you have ever had the experience of still loving and caring for something, even in a moment of anger or hatred, you understand that it is possible to be compassionate toward something even when you don't like it. Can you try to apply the same to yourself? To treat yourself as you would treat the child or puppy? There may be parts that you don't like, but are you able to hold on to a fundamental sense of care for yourself, of wanting the best for yourself, even if you don't like what is happening in that moment?

One path to increased self-compassion is through gratitude or "self-appreciation," the act of being thankful for the good that lives in all of us.[10] Many of us (especially those raised as girls) are socialized to focus on the things that we don't like about ourselves, to criticize ourselves, and tear ourselves down. We are presented with impossible benchmarks to meet, and then blame ourselves for our perceived imperfections. In some ways this can feel protective; if we criticize ourselves, we beat others to the punch. No one can tell us how much we suck when we are already telling it to ourselves. Giving ourselves a compliment can feel vulnerable, like we are letting our guard down and giving someone a chance to sucker punch us. We imagine that others will snicker at our pride; *I can't believe she thinks she looks good in that, what a fool!* To avoid this, we tend to be intensely hard on ourselves, manifested both in the way we speak to ourselves (i.e., our inner critic) and the way that we speak about ourselves to others (i.e., self-deprecating humor, difficulty accepting a compliment, and other forms of putting ourselves down). While it may feel safer to be self-critical, this constant berating takes a toll on our mental health.

In contrast, focusing on the things that you like about yourself is linked with enhanced psychological well-being, warm relationships with others, increased self-acceptance, personal growth, and a greater sense of purpose in life.[11] One study found that writing about things you appreciate about your body was associated with improved body image and less weight bias internalization.[12] Pause here for a moment and think about at least one thing that you feel grateful for about your body. What do you like about your body? What do you appreciate? Perhaps it is your strong legs that bring you where you need to go, your gut that helps you break down your food so your body has the energy to thrive, or simply the fact that you are breathing and alive.

Along with self-compassion, acceptance is a powerful tool in quieting our inner critic and disrupting disordered cycles around food and body. Acceptance is the process of perceiving and acknowledging your experience rather than judging it as good or bad. It is simply about opening our eyes to the reality of our current situation, right here, in this very moment. Rather than fighting against reality, acceptance is about tuning in to our current experience and acknowledging it without judgment.

Acceptance is founded on "nonjudgmental observation," a process of noticing, describing, and approaching things as they truly are in the current moment, without the narratives and evaluations that we usually superimpose on our experiences. For example, if we walk into our dining room to find a piece of chocolate cake on the table, we may ordinarily think, *Wow, that looks delicious, I want to eat the whole thing, but I shouldn't have any cake, once I start eating something like that I won't be able to control myself, I'm trying to stick to being good today and that means no sugar, maybe one bite won't hurt, no, it's too fattening, I really shouldn't, who bought that cake, is someone trying to sabotage my diet, why is my partner always so insensitive, I can't stand them!* With all the baggage that we are bringing to the table (pun intended), the mere sight of the cake has sent our anxiety through the roof! Now if we were to encounter the same cake while practicing nonjudgmental observation, we may simply describe it as brown, shiny in places, spongy textured, and triangular shaped. We may notice the sensations that arise in our body upon encountering the cake: salivation starting in our mouth, grumbles in our tummy, increased heartbeat and pulse, rapid breathing. In this scenario, the cake isn't good or bad—it just is.

It is human nature to make judgments and create stories around our experiences. It is how we organize and make sense of the world. Judgment serves an important role; for example, if you come across a poisonous tarantula spider, you don't want to nonjudgmentally observe this creature as brown, hairy, and eight-legged and get up close for a better look. You want to judge it as dangerous and get as far away from it as possible. When it comes to judging our food choices, our bodies, and ourselves, however, judgments are far less useful. Judgments distort the reality of the current moment. They make us see things through the lens of what we believe them to be, not what they truly are. We overlay stories from our past, creating an obscured view of the present. It keeps us stuck in diet culture by labeling foods as good or bad, permitted or restricted, and on the wagon or off the wagon. It also keeps us mired in self-hatred when we judge ourselves as good or bad—and we tend to be more judgmental of ourselves than others. Harsh judgments about ourselves can make us feel miserable and stuck in entrenched patterns. Working toward observing our eating, our body, and ourselves with a sense of nonjudgmental awareness can help us change our harsh critical stance with ourselves.

Practicing mindfulness and cultivating nonjudgmental awareness do not mean that we will never make judgments. Rather, the intention is to simply become more aware of the judgments that we are making. Awareness can transform judgment to discernment. While judgment labels things as good or bad, wanted or not wanted, okay or not okay, discernment enables us to make choices with attunement to our unique needs in the present moment. Discernment involves evaluating the different options available at any given moment and choosing the one that is the best fit. For example, with the cake that we spoke about earlier, discernment may include checking in with your body, assessing if you are hungry or not, whether you want the cake now or later or not at all, whether this particular cake looks appealing, and how you may feel after eating the cake, eventually leading you to make a choice about whether or not you want to eat the cake. There is no right or wrong answer, just different options based on what works best for you at that moment.

I want to emphasize here that the intention is not to eliminate all judgments from your mind, but rather to gently observe the judgments that will inevitably arise and to shift the way that you relate to these thoughts. As I said before, it's human nature to judge things—especially ourselves! It is a tough habit to break free from, and we are never going to live our entire lives in a judgment-free zone—nor would we want to. It's usually not long after learning about acceptance and nonjudgmental awareness that people start berating themselves for being judgmental. *I don't know what is wrong with me, I can't stop judging myself, I'm such a failure.* The irony of judging our judgments is not lost. If you notice yourself being judgmental, remember that *this* is the moment of awareness, *this* is the very practice that you are cultivating, and thank your mind for offering you the gift of awareness. Know that to be human is to be judgmental, and try your best to meet your judgments with compassion.

How can I accept myself if I don't like myself? Won't acceptance mean that I'm giving up? These are some of the concerns that make people bristle at the idea of acceptance. Many of us believe that acceptance means liking something, being okay with it, or that it will stay that way forever. To address these concerns, it is important to remember a few things about acceptance. Acceptance has nothing to do with liking. It is simply about observing our experience without judgment and clearly facing reality. Acceptance has nothing to do with the future. It is just about the present moment. Accepting things as they are in this moment doesn't mean that things will stay the same. In fact, things never stay the same. That is the nature of time—it is always moving forward, and the present moment is always changing. We can accept that something is the way that it is right now, have self-compassion, dislike it, and want it to change all at the same time.

We tend to believe that if we don't look at something it will just go away. If we talk about it, we will make it worse. Let's take teen pregnancy as an example. For a long time, people have fought against comprehensive sex education with the argument that if you teach teens about sex, it will give them the idea to go out and do it. Yet we see that areas without sex education have higher rates of teen pregnancy. This is an example of denial, or the belief that if we don't look at something it's not really happening. When we face something head-on (e.g., accept the fact that teens are having sex, with or without education), we can look at the reality of the current situation (acceptance) and figure out the best way forward. In the case of teen pregnancy, research suggests that providing comprehensive sex education can reduce the risk of pregnancy by 60 percent.[13] Accepting what is happening allows us to move forward from where we are now, not live in denial wishing we were somewhere else.

Imagine that you accidentally fall into a flowing river. In a panic you realize you need to get out of the water and furiously start trying to swim upstream, toward where you fell in. Quickly you find that fighting against the flow of the river is an exhausting and futile endeavor. Too tired to keep struggling, you discover that you can swim along with the current with relative ease, and eventually the river flow brings you to a spot where you can easily come ashore and walk back to where you need to be. In this example, the downstream-flowing river is the reality of what is happening at the present moment in your life. You can't change it, because it is already happening. But you can choose whether to respond with acceptance or with denial. You can either swim with the river and "go with the flow" (acceptance) or you can struggle and exhaust yourself trying to fight the current (denial). Neither acceptance nor denial changes the reality of the moment. Either way, you are still in the river.

When we stop fighting against reality and accept what is happening in the current moment, we can make conscious choices about how we want to move forward in our life. And we can choose to do so with compassion. In contrast, when we are in denial, we stay stuck on autopilot, being a passive passenger on the ride of life.

After several months of treatment, Tracy described her process of acceptance as follows: "All of these years I felt like a caged bird. I've been stuck in this trap, desperately flapping my wings to get out. Everything I've been doing to try and make myself better—the dieting, the binge eating, the plans to start a new life-changing weight loss program on Monday—it's all just been flapping my wings. I'm exhausted and still stuck in this damn cage. When I started practicing acceptance, the first step was realizing that I've been stuck in a cage and flapping my wings really isn't helping get me out. Initially I thought that acceptance was just about settling into life in the cage and trying to be content eating my seed and swinging from my perch. But once I stopped frantically flapping around and settled onto my perch, I saw what acceptance was really about. Centered on my perch, I was suddenly able to see the bars that I had been flapping up against. And more importantly, I was able to see that those bars weren't fixed; some of them made up a door, and I could easily see my way out of the cage. Acceptance isn't about giving up and living in the cage; acceptance is about freedom."

Here are a few more examples of statements of denial and compassionate acceptance to help clarify:

Denial: It's not okay for my body to weigh this much.

Acceptance: This is the weight that my body currently is. How can I care for myself now in the best ways possible with compassion?

Denial: Once I lose weight, I'll start dating.

Acceptance: How can I work toward my goal of dating now, in my current body? How can I address the negative feelings I have about my body today that stop me from fully engaging in my life? How can I be as happy as possible now, while I am single? Do I want a partner, or is that just something I've believed I need to have in my life to be valuable?

Denial: My pants are too tight and uncomfortable, but I'm not going to buy new clothes because I should be able to fit into these pants.

Acceptance: I'll wear pants that fit my current body, so I can be comfortable now.

Do you ever listen to the internal dialogue in your head? For most of us, this is not a friendly conversation. Just as Tracy had an inner bully berating her day in and day out, so do many of us. We say cruel things to ourselves that we wouldn't dream of saying to anyone else. It's like a tape recording of someone telling us that we suck, playing all day long.

Are you ready to change the tape? The "golden rule" teaches us to treat others as we want to be treated. But for most of us, the opposite is the real challenge: treat yourself as you would treat someone else. Recognizing this voice and bringing it into full awareness is the first step to change. Mindfulness allows us to observe our inner dialogue while creating the space and distance we need to consciously respond to it.

If you've been practicing the daily mindfulness meditation that we learned in chapter 3, you may already be more aware of your internal dialogue. You may have noticed it during your meditation practice when your mind wandered off and you harshly reprimanded yourself. Or when you judged yourself for not meditating enough or not doing it right. You may have noticed critical thoughts about your body during meditations, perhaps the discomfort of your belly hanging over your pants when you sit or the way the inner sides of your arms press against the side of your body. Consider the moments when this dialogue enters your full awareness to be a gift; that is your invitation to change.

When you notice this harsh inner voice, the first step is to label it. You can simply label it "inner bully" or "inner critic." Some people find it helpful to give this voice an actual name, like "Ruby" or "Bill." (No offense to any Rubys or Bills out there!) You may even find it helpful to imagine this voice as a little creature—can you visualize it? Just pick something that resonates for you and go with it.

Labeling this voice helps us get some distance from it and see that it's not the truth. It is just your thoughts, internalizations from a culture that teaches us from the youngest ages that there is something wrong with our body. These thoughts are mere activities of our mind; they are not a gospel that we need to live by. With practice and time, we can replace our inner bully with an inner kind companion who can accompany us on the path away from dieting and self-hatred.

Once you have labeled the voice, practice acknowledging it (*there is my harsh critical voice* or *hello, Ruby*). Then allow that voice to shift from the forefront of your mind to the background by bringing your full awareness to something that is happening now, like your breath. Our intention is to shift this voice to the background rather than eliminate it altogether. Ironically, when we focus on getting rid of something, we can spend a lot of time and energy fighting against it. We don't want to get locked in a power battle trying to get rid of the voice—because remember, when we fight against ourselves, we always lose. When we can accept that the voice is there, we can choose where we want to focus our attention and how we want to respond to this voice.

When you have recognized the voice, labeled it, and shifted your attention to the present moment (by focusing on your breath), you can pause and ask yourself:

- How can I best take care of myself in this moment?
- What do I truly need?
- How can I treat myself with kindness and compassion?

It is natural to keep getting pulled back to your inner critic. That voice is strong and is used to being the center of attention. You can go through this process as many times as necessary. It is not uncommon for you to notice your inner critic, label it, shift your awareness to focus on your breath, but hardly a minute later notice that you have gotten caught back up listening to your inner critic. As always, be gentle with yourself. When this happens, without judgment simply start anew with noticing your inner critic, labeling, refocusing, and so on.

Just like you are learning to be your own kind companion, so did Tracy. Along with the other group participants, Tracy practiced mindful eating and made the trip to my office in midtown Manhattan every Wednesday evening to participate in the group. In her day-to-day life, Tracy kept herself very busy. When she wasn't juggling the schedules of her two kids, grocery shopping, caring for the house, prepping dinner, helping with homework, and taking their dog for a walk, she was zoned out to Netflix. Her time at my office was one of the rare moments when she allowed herself to slow down and be quiet with her own thoughts.

I led a guided meditation to start the group. "Notice your breath as it enters and exits your body, bringing your full awareness to the breath as you inhale and as you exhale."

Tracy tried to focus on her breath but kept becoming distracted by the way that the waist of her too-small pants dug into her belly. When she sat down, she could really feel it. That sent her inner bully into action. *What the hell is wrong with you! Now you've really done it; you've eaten your way out of these pants. You have absolutely no self-control. You are disgusting. Everyone is probably laughing at you and how your belly is billowing out. You are such a loser.*

I noticed the tension in Tracy's face and tried to guide her back. "If you notice that your mind has wandered off, gently, lovingly see where it's gone, and bring your awareness back to your breath."

Tracy realized, *Oh, brother, Tim's taken over!* She had labeled her inner bully Tim, in homage to her pediatrician from all those years back. *Hello, Tim.* Tracy labeled these thoughts with a greeting. Next she shifted her awareness to the present moment. As she brought her breath into the forefront of her mind, the critical voice of Tim naturally shifted to the background. The voice was still there, but it was much quieter. She focused on her breath for another minute or so, noticing as Tim got louder again, when she would again label it and shift back to her breath.

When I rang the meditation bell to signal the end of the practice, Tracy had a new awareness of just how incessant her critical voice was. After the meditation, she shared her experience observing, labeling, and shifting her inner bully to the background of her mind while focusing on her breath. I said, "Thank you for sharing that, Tracy. What a wonderful new insight! But don't forget the last step: self-compassion. How can you move forward with compassion?"

Tracy thought for a moment. "Well, I guess I could start by buying new pants that actually fit my current body." It was such a simple and, in many ways, mundane solution—clothes shopping—but at the same time quite revolutionary.

Now that you've learned the steps involved in quieting your inner critic, how can you implement these tools to become your own kind companion? How can you respond to yourself with compassion instead of cruelty?

TAKE-ACTION ACTIVITIES

Be self-compassionate

Listen to the guided audio meditation on self-compassion at www .drconason.com/diet-free-revolution/. Research suggests that listening to a twenty-minute self-compassion meditation daily for three weeks is associated with significant improvements in body image. Try it and see if you notice a difference!

Try this body gratitude exercise that helped improve body image and reduce internalized weight bias in a research study.[14] Think about aspects of your body that you are grateful for. This can be anything, including your health, physical appearance, or the functionality of your body. Try to come up with at least five things. Take a minute and really think about those things, picturing them in your mind. Once you have finished thinking about those things, choose at least three of them and write about why you are grateful for those things.

Set the intention of doing at least one kind act for yourself this week, something that makes you feel loved and cared for. It could be planning a dinner date with yourself to your favorite restaurant, carving out time to mindfully listen to your favorite song (and maybe even dance to it), getting a massage, or saying no to a project you don't want to take on. Make it a priority to complete your act of kindness, and don't let anything get in your way.

Practice quieting your inner critic

You can notice and minimize a critical internal voice by using a four-step process:

1. Increase **awareness** of your inner voice through mindfulness practice.

2. **Label** the voice (e.g., "inner critic" or "Ruby").

3. **Shift** awareness to the present moment (e.g., focus on breath).

4. Move forward with **compassion**.

Maintain your mindfulness

Continue to practice the mindfulness of breath meditation for five minutes per day, either using the guided meditation available at www .drconason.com/diet-free-revolution/ or setting a timer for five minutes and leading yourself through the practice of focusing on your breath, noticing when your mind has wandered off, and gently bringing your awareness back to your breath (see chapter 3 for more instructions on the mindfulness of breath practice).

Continue to use the mindful pause to check in with your body prior to meals and throughout the day (see chapter 3 for more instructions on the mindful pause).

5

STEP 5: Hear and Feed Your Hunger

Michael came to see me at the request of Sue Sherman, his long-time therapist, who I had trained with at a community mental health clinic. Sue now specializes in treating depression and had worked with Michael for a couple of years, making good headway on improving his mood. Over the previous few months, however, Michael's disordered eating had come into the forefront, and she'd realized he needed more targeted eating disorder treatment.

"He's an interesting guy," Sue had told me on the phone, after obtaining Michael's permission to speak with me about his treatment. "Many people would see him as a success story. He's lost a lot of weight—and I really mean *a lot*—and he is incredibly self-disciplined in sticking to his program. But sometimes he has these episodes where he completely goes off the rails. He is obsessed with food, both eating it and not eating it. And the amount of time he spends at the gym! It's shut out everything else in his life."

I'd agreed to a consultation session with Michael, and less than a week later we were sitting together in my office. Michael was a tall man with a notable physical presence; he was dressed casually in a sporty matching sweatsuit and carried an enormous coffee in with him. The size of the coffee seemed proportional to his stature. He sat in the club chair catty-corner to mine, forcing me to reposition my chair to face him directly. Few people choose to sit in this chair. The couch is far more inviting, positioned in the center of the room directly across from my reclining chair, with an end table next to it with a box of tissues and a coaster for people to put a drink on. The chair Michael was sitting in was further away from me, almost at the other end of the room. Perhaps he felt more comfortable with distance or wished to avoid literally being on a therapist's couch. Or maybe he just preferred chairs to couches. After all, as Sigmund Freud famously said, "Sometimes a cigar is just a cigar."

Michael relaxed into the chair, stretching out his legs to utilize the full depth of the seat. He let out a sigh as he precariously balanced the enormous coffee on the thick upholstered arm of the chair. He nervously bounced one leg up and down in a motion that I was sure would spill his coffee all over my carpeted floor.

"I'm not exactly sure why I'm here," Michael started out. "Things are pretty much okay." But as he started to explain his situation to me, it sounded anything but okay.

Michael was twenty-three years old and lived alone in a studio apartment. His pet ferret, Buddy, was his one constant companion. He found solace in Buddy, a creature who loved him unconditionally. People were far more fickle. Michael grew up as a fat kid and learned firsthand how cruel people can be. Starting in middle school, Michael was rarely called by his first name. Instead, kids called him "Klump," after the character Sherman Klump from the film *The Nutty Professor*, played by Eddie Murphy in a fat suit, where the punch line of the comedy was the character's weight. He had hoped that he would be able to escape the teasing when he started at a new high school, but alas Sean Miller, the popular captain of the basketball team and class A bully, also moved from Michael's middle school to the same high school. It was hardly mid-September before he started hearing the familiar refrain "Hey Plump Klump!" yelled at him in the hallways. He went through high school with his head down, doing everything in his power to go unnoticed. He wore clothes that were unobtrusive, rarely spoke in class, and tried to shrink himself in every way possible.

The summer after Michael graduated high school, he started the process of bariatric weight loss surgery. At his first visit to the surgery center, he found himself in a room full of other fat people, all desperate to rid themselves of their fatness. They sat in a conference room on folding chairs and watched a video that described the different surgical procedures, the recovery process, and the strict diet they would have to follow. Michael sat through it all, but all he could focus on was the woman who had undergone the surgery who came to talk to the group. Michael couldn't believe it: she was thin! In a dramatic fashion, she pulled a pair of old jeans out from a shopping bag and gleefully stepped with both feet into one leg, pulling the pant leg up to her waist, the spare leg flailing like a wind sock flag in the breeze. "Now I'm half the size! If I can do it, you can too!" she said with encouragement. That was all Michael needed to hear. He didn't care what it would take—he would have this surgery. It was his only hope. Before the summer was over, Michael was back at the surgery center to have part of his stomach removed and his digestive tract rerouted in a gastric bypass surgery.

This will be a new start, he promised himself.

In the years that followed, Michael dedicated his life to counting every calorie, tracking every step, following a strict diet, going to the gym for hours every single day, critiquing his image in the mirror each morning, and weighing himself incessantly. His activity tracker was omnipresent. If he didn't meet his daily number of steps, he would walk around the block late at night until the little device on his wrist turned green, indicating that he had met his goal for the day, sometimes just minutes before the device reset at midnight.

Michael worked as a fourth-grade teacher, which he found rewarding but which came second to his true "passion" for maintaining his weight. While the pay wasn't great, he liked that he got out of work early enough to make it to the gym before the evening rush, allowing him to commandeer an elliptical machine before the forty-five-minute time limit set in at 6 p.m. Summer break meant "beast mode" as he called it, when, without the time commitment of going to work, he could follow his meal plan even more religiously and tack on an extra hour to his already-extensive gym routine.

Weight loss had left Michael with large flaps of skin hanging like a deflated balloon around his body. Vestiges of his former life. Each morning he went through an elaborate ritual using elastic bandages and compression garments to bind himself, so the hanging skin wouldn't be visible under his clothes. Throughout the day, the bandages constricted him and made it uncomfortable to sit, a constant reminder of how his body betrayed him. He used this as "motivation" to eat as little as possible during the day. His childhood memories of being Plump Klump were never far from the surface. He was terrified to date, convinced no one could ever be attracted to him. At school when he heard a group of kids laughing, he immediately tensed up. *Are they laughing at me?* he wondered. *You are not Plump Klump anymore,* he reminded himself several times a day. He's never sure if he really believed it.

Recently Michael's rigid adherence to his "healthy lifestyle" (his words, not mine) had gotten a little less rigid. Namely, he was starting to binge. This terrified him, not only because he hated feeling out of control, but also because it meant the gastric bypass surgery wasn't restricting his eating anymore. While the procedure had initially forced him to eat child-sized meals of specific permissible foods, this was no longer the case. He could eat like he did before surgery. And if the surgery wasn't restricting his eating anymore, what was stopping him from becoming Plump Klump again? The thought sent chills down his spine.

Each day when Michael came home from the gym, he would make himself a dinner of grilled chicken breast with steamed broccoli. Sometimes he alternated with a piece of grilled salmon and steamed cauliflower. One day a few months prior, after reading an article that named sweet potatoes the latest superfood, he had baked one to go along with his dinner. Afterward the guilt was overwhelming. Sweet potatoes have carbs and sugar. Before he knew it, he was in a full-on spiral, feeling like he had lost control of his eating and blown his diet. In a fugue-like state, he put his coat over his house clothes and, still wearing his slippers, made his way down to the bodega on his corner, where he bought all his childhood favorites. Little Debbie snack cakes, mac and cheese in the box, candy bars, and ice cream.

He went back to his apartment and ate most of it before he could even take off his coat. Then, disgusted with himself, still wearing his coat, he took the remaining food out to the curb and threw it in the trash outside his building. Mystified, he came back home and tried to make sense of what had happened. How could he have lost control like that? All he knew was that he couldn't allow it to happen again.

But happen again it did. It wasn't more than a week before a similar episode ensued, and then another one a few days after that. Michael worried that the thinner life he had worked so diligently to uphold was slipping away like grains of sand through his fingers.

Michael blamed himself for binge eating, believing that if he could just resist his temptations, the problem would go away. But as I listened to Michael describe his restrictive eating, it became clear that the problem wasn't his discipline or willpower; the problem was his hunger—or more accurately, his disconnection from his hunger. As Michael recounted the sparse amount of food he subsisted on for most of the day, I had one thought: *he must be starving.*

We are taught that hunger is something to be suppressed and subdued. The old Lap-Band (a bariatric-surgery device) advertisement is a clear example of how the weight loss industry demonizes hunger. The ad, which aired in 2006, personified hunger as a fierce lion roaring while a woman stands nearby describing how her hunger told her to "eat, eat, eat." That is, until she undergoes bariatric surgery, which finally allows her to tame her hunger, now transformed from the vicious lion into a docile tabby cat, snuggling sweetly on her lap. Clearly, taming our hunger is something to be desired. Tips to curb your hunger abound, ranging from the ineffective but relatively benign, like drinking more water or eating more fiber, to potentially fatal, like eating cotton balls (please don't try that at home—or anywhere else!). Appetite-suppressant pills are widely available (with no age restrictions) over the counter at your local drugstore, and ads featuring celebrities target kids and teens with products like appetite-suppressant lollipops.

The truth is that there is only one good appetite suppressant—food. Our body's hunger signals guide us to nourish our body. They help us know when to eat and when we've had enough. When we eat food, miraculously our hunger signals subside. Eating is the only appetite suppressant our body was designed for. When we try to trick our body by artificially suppressing our hunger or ignoring the signals our body is sending us, we can dysregulate our entire appetite system. In this chapter we are going to learn how to hear our hunger signals and eat to satisfy them, so we can use this important signal to guide our eating rather than fight against our own survival mechanisms.

The Physiology of Hunger

Our body comes equipped with a sophisticated hunger-response system to help us know when to start eating and when we've had enough to eat. It is like a coordinated dance between our organs, hormones, nutrient stores, and brain. When our stomach has been empty for approximately two hours, it starts contracting to push any food remnants into our intestines. This is called "borborygmus," and it's what is happening when we hear our tummy grumbling. Concurrently, the cells in our stomach and intestines produce the hormone ghrelin (remember the "hunger hormone" we learned about in chapter 1?), which lets our brain know that it's time to eat. As ghrelin increases, leptin, the "satiety hormone" secreted by our fat cells, decreases in response to the depletion of nutrients stored in our body fat and liver. This decrease in leptin also signals the hypothalamus that we need food. The vagus nerve, which serves as a direct connection between our digestive system and our brain, carries information about how empty or full our stomach is and tells our brain how much nutrients are in our intestines. When our brain receives this cacophony of signals from ghrelin, leptin, and the vagus nerve, it releases neurotransmitters including neuropeptide Y, which stimulates our appetite and tells us to seek out food. It also triggers the stomach to release gastric acids to prepare for digestion.

Glucose, a type of sugar, is our brain's fuel. It's what our brain needs to function properly. When we are nourished, our brain can get the glucose it needs by breaking down the food we eat. Carbohydrates are our body's preferred macronutrient to break down into glucose, but it can also use protein or fat in a pinch. When we don't eat in response to hunger, our brain doesn't have the glucose it needs to run optimally, and we start to feel it. This is why we can get "hangry," or irritable, when we don't eat in response to hunger. We can also feel tired and weak, be more impulsive, have difficulty concentrating, have trouble making long-term decisions, and feel shaky and sweaty. As our hunger grows and we don't eat, our body starts to perceive that we are in threat of starvation, a life-threatening situation. The brain sends signals to our organs and hormones to increase blood glucose levels through alternative mechanisms reserved for times of crisis. This causes the adrenal gland to produce the stress hormones cortisol and adrenaline, which trigger the "fight-or-flight" response. In survival mode, our brain signals for us to seek out the most readily available foods that will raise our blood sugar, particularly carbohydrates and simple sugars that can easily be broken down into glucose to get our brain the fuel it needs. When we get to this extreme point of hunger, our body is in panic mode and our eating may feel frantic or out of control.

There has been a lot of research into how our hunger-response system can be manipulated. Ghrelin and leptin have been of interest to the pharmaceutical industry for quite some time. Certain bariatric-surgery procedures like Roux-en-Y gastric bypass surgery alter the gut hormones by cutting away organ tissue from the stomach and intestines. There have even been procedures to freeze the vagus nerve! But at the end of the day, if any of this was effective long-term, it would be widely used. With the possible exception of certain bariatric-surgery procedures—which come with significant risks—we are not able to change our body's natural hunger-response system. Which is a testament to how wise and powerful our body truly is.

Navigating with Our Internal GPS: Hunger

Our hunger-response system does a great job at letting us know when it's time to eat. The problem is, we often don't listen to it. When we've spent so much of our life disconnected from our hunger and mistrusting our body, it may be hard to hear the hunger signals that our body is sending us. Do you know when you are hungry?

Let's try this brief exercise. Sit with your feet flat on the ground, your hips slightly higher than your knees, and your spine upright. If this position is not comfortable or accessible for you, take whatever position your body is calling for. Focus on your breath for a few breath cycles. Notice the sensation of your breath as it enters and exits your body; bring your full awareness to your body in the present moment. Now focus your awareness on your belly. Are you aware of any sensations of hunger? How do you know this? What physical sensations do you notice? Whatever you noticed (or didn't notice), take note because we'll be returning to it later in this chapter. And don't worry if you couldn't identify any sensations of hunger—that's what we are here to learn about!

The Hunger Scale is a tool that can help you identify your hunger. We often think of hunger as an on-off experience: either we are hungry, or we are not. But hunger exists on a spectrum, and there are many gradations we miss when we think of it as a dichotomous yes-or-no experience. The Hunger Scale was designed to help you capture the range of different hunger experiences. Rather than asking *if* you are hungry, the Hunger Scale prompts you to think about *how* hungry you are.

Hunger builds slowly over time. As hunger progresses, sensations change and intensify. The Hunger Scale ranges from 0 to 4, with 0 being least hungry and 4 being most hungry. Physiological sensations of hunger can vary from person to person. It is important for you to tune in to your unique experience of hunger. I encourage you to go to www.drconason .com/diet-free-revolution/ to download a blank Hunger Scale and complete the scale with the sensations of hunger that you experience. You will find a completed Hunger Scale with commonly experienced sensations of hunger on the next page. I'm going to review some of these common sensations, but please don't let me become another expert telling you what your body is supposed to experience! Always prioritize the information coming from your own body and honor your unique signals, which may be different from what I describe here.

On the Hunger Scale, a 0 indicates the absence of hunger signals. When you are not hungry, you may feel full or you may feel satiated (neither hungry nor full). We are going to be learning about fullness in the next chapter, so for now just think of a 0 as the lack of hunger sensations.

If you are paying close attention to your bodily sensations, you may notice the start of hunger, represented by a 1 on the Hunger Scale. These are the mildest sensations of hunger and may include a slight gentle grumbling in your stomach, churning of the stomach acids, or a feeling of emptiness in your stomach. It can be helpful to place your hand on your stomach (located on the left side of your upper abdomen) to help you focus your attention to this part of the body and see if you notice any sensations.

HUNGER SCALE

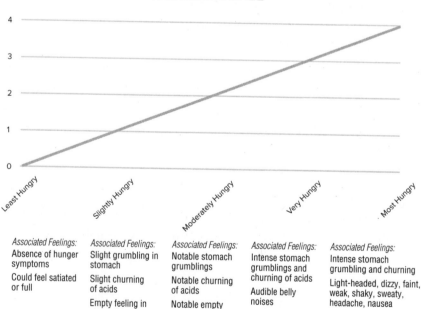

	Least Hungry	Slightly Hungry	Moderately Hungry	Very Hungry	Most Hungry
Associated Feelings:	Absence of hunger symptoms	Slight grumbling in stomach	Notable stomach grumblings	Intense stomach grumblings and churning of acids	Intense stomach grumbling and churning
	Could feel satiated or full	Slight churning of acids	Notable churning of acids	Audible belly noises	Light-headed, dizzy, faint, weak, shaky, sweaty, headache, nausea
		Empty feeling in stomach	Notable empty feeling in stomach	Drop in blood sugar	Low blood sugar

If you don't eat in response to these early mild symptoms, your hunger will progress to a 2 on the Hunger Scale. Here you may experience more moderate hunger sensations including more significant stomach grumbling, more notable churning of the stomach acids, and definite feelings of emptiness in the stomach.

If you don't eat in response to these more moderate sensations of hunger, your hunger will continue to progress and you will feel very hungry, designated by a 3 on the Hunger Scale. When you are very hungry, you may feel intense sensations of grumbling in your stomach that may even be audible to other people, as well as significant churning of the stomach acids. At this point your hunger is hard to ignore. It may be difficult to think about anything but eating as thoughts of food intrude into whatever else you are doing. You may experience low blood sugar and associated symptoms like irritability, difficulty focusing, a headache, shakiness, and fatigue.

If you still don't eat in response to your hunger, you will progress to most hungry, denoted by a 4 on the Hunger Scale. At this point your body is going into crisis mode, desperately sending out signals for you to eat. You may experience intense audible stomach grumblings and acid churning; the symptoms of low blood sugar may give you a headache or make you feel light-headed, dizzy, faint, weak, shaky, trembling, sweaty, or nauseous. You likely feel preoccupied with thoughts about eating and feel driven to seek out food, especially carbohydrates and sugars, which your body can readily break down into glucose. These sensations are nearly impossible to ignore, and most people feel uncomfortable when they reach this end of the scale.

The Hunger Scale focuses on the physiological signs of hunger. These are the physical sensations that occur in our belly and tend to be our most reliable indicators of hunger. In addition to the grumbling, churning, and feelings of emptiness in our stomach, we may also notice non-belly signs of hunger such as increased thoughts of foods, more cravings for food, tiredness, irritability, and difficulty focusing. I recommend using the belly sensations (if you can identify them) as the primary source of information because these signals are unique. It is unusual to experience sensations like stomach grumbling and churning acids when we don't feel hungry. But we often feel tired, irritable, or distracted, and think of food at times when we are not physiologically hungry. These symptoms can be useful when used in concert with the belly sensations; for example, stomach rumblings, acid churning, thoughts of food, and irritability paint a clear picture of hunger. That being said, the most important thing is that you trust the hunger signs that are most salient for you, whether they be belly signs or non-belly signs.

Remember the mindful pause exercise that we learned about in chapter 3? Now that we've learned about hunger, we can use the mindful pause to tune in to our hunger throughout the day. A mindful pause for hunger is like the exercise noticing our belly sensations we did earlier in this chapter, but now we can use the Hunger Scale to identify hunger. A mindful pause for hunger involves the following:

1. Assume the meditative position, seated with your spine upright and your feet flat on the ground, or whatever position your body is calling for.

2. Bring your full awareness to your breath for three or four breath cycles.

3. Expand your awareness to focus on your stomach. Do you notice any sensations of hunger? How hungry are you? Give yourself a rating between 0 (absence of hunger) and 4 (most hungry). How did you decide on your rating? What sensations informed your decision?

You may notice yourself using external factors to decide how hungry you feel. For example, *I'm a 3 on the Hunger Scale because it's been a few hours since I last ate.* Or *I'm a 2 because it's 12:30 p.m. and I always eat lunch at this time; if it's lunchtime I must be hungry.* These external cues are not as reliable because they are not attuned to your internal experiences. You may not be hungry at lunchtime. Relying on external cues can make you second-guess your internal hunger signals. For example, if you find your stomach grumbling but you just ate an hour earlier, you may think,

I can't possibly be hungry, I just ate. I'll let you in on a secret here: you can be hungry even if you just ate, especially if what you ate wasn't satisfying. Mindful eating is all about prioritizing the messages from your own body above the ones from the outside environment. As much as you can, try to trust what your body is telling you.

When you identify physiological hunger, by default you also identify emotional drives to eat. For the purposes of this book, we categorize any eating that is not driven by physiological hunger as emotional eating. It's a broad category. We'll do a deep dive into emotional eating in chapter 9, but for now I want you to know that emotional eating is a healthy part of normal unconflicted eating. Think about it: if we only ate when physiologically hungry, who would ever eat dessert after a full meal? What a sad world that would be. There is a villainization of emotional eating because, in our fatphobic puritanical culture, we are programmed to believe that it is virtuous to eat as little as possible; eating should only serve the most utilitarian purposes. This is evident in the popular "food is fuel" mantra. Food isn't just fuel—it is also a form of connection with others, with our cultural identity, a source of relaxation, pleasure, and enjoyment. These aspects of eating are essential to our well-being and are very much part of a healthy, balanced way of eating. This book isn't advocating the eat-only-when-hungry diet. If you try to turn it into that, it will backfire. Because diets don't work, remember?

The purpose of focusing on physiological hunger is to make sure you are eating enough and that you are nourishing your body in accordance with its natural signals. If you are someone who struggles with overeating or binge eating, it may seem odd to think about making sure you eat enough. You may think, *Of course I'm eating enough—in fact, I'm eating too much!* We are far more likely to conceptualize the "problem" as eating too much. But "overeating" is almost always paired with restriction, whether it be physically not eating enough or a restrictive mindset where we judge our eating and believe that food will become scarce. You may skip meals or go long periods of time without food or with eating very little, only to find yourself feeling out of control around food later in the day. Because we live in a culture where undereating is seen as virtuous and overeating is gluttonous, we tend to categorize the times that we have half a grapefruit for breakfast or skip lunch as moments when we are "successful" and the time that we ate an entire pizza pie as the problem. But the two are inextricably linked, different sides of the same coin. Restriction is what fuels cycles of overeating/binge eating, and that is the first place to intervene. Adequately nourishing your body lays the foundation for healing your relationship with food.

Still Can't Identify Hunger?

If you are having difficulty identifying hunger, here are a few other experiments to try. Delay eating after you wake up in the morning. Instead of eating breakfast at your usual time, check in with your hunger. If you don't feel any sensations of hunger (a 0 rating on the Hunger Scale), wait a bit before eating. Use this time to "watch" your belly sensations, checking in with yourself to see if any signs of hunger arise. Don't get distracted doing something else; you want to make sure that you are checking in with your hunger at least every fifteen minutes or so. Be sure to have food available, so that when you notice your hunger emerge and reach a comfortable level, you can satisfy it. If your hunger hasn't emerged in a few hours, eat and try this exercise again another time.

It can also help to eliminate any artificial appetite suppressants from your diet. Caffeine tends to be the biggest culprit here. If you are having trouble identifying hunger and you subsist on coffee or energy drinks for large portions of your day, experiment with switching to a decaffeinated beverage, or at least reducing your caffeine intake, and see if your hunger starts to emerge. Certain medications can also affect appetite; if you are on a medication that suppresses your appetite, discuss this with your medical provider.

If you have tried delaying eating and eliminating appetite suppressants and you still haven't been able to identify any signs of hunger, you can try to invite out your hunger signals with more structured eating. This may be especially useful if you tend to go long periods of time without eating. When we habitually don't nourish our body, our hunger cues can get dysregulated. Feeding your body balanced meals and snacks with enough nutrients at regular intervals—every two to four hours—can help recalibrate your hunger signals. You may experiment with eating in this structured way for a few weeks and see if your hunger signals return. Working with a weight-inclusive, Health at Every Size–informed dietitian can be helpful in this process.

If you have tried these suggestions and are still unable to experience any sensations of hunger, it is recommended that you consult with your health care provider to rule out any medical issues that may be contributing to your lack of hunger. And as a reminder, if you are struggling with an eating disorder, work with a treatment team to evaluate if the strategies in this book are appropriate for your treatment at this time.

Satisfy Your Hunger

Now that you are getting familiar with the experience of hunger in your body, the next step is to eat when you are hungry. It may sound basic, but when we've had a long-standing conflicted relationship with food, it can be hard to do.

As you begin your mindful eating adventure, you may wonder: *When do I start eating? How hungry should I be?* There is no universal "right" place on the Hunger Scale to begin eating. It is a process of experimentation to see where *you* feel most comfortable. Some people like to eat as soon as they notice hunger emerge, around a 1 on the scale, while others prefer to let their hunger build a bit more before eating, waiting until a 2 or 3 on the scale. Most people feel uncomfortable at the upper end of the Hunger Scale at a 3 or 4. Try starting to eat at various points on the scale, and explore what feels best for you. You may choose to mark your Hunger Scale with a star or other notation next to the point(s) where you like to eat. But remember, this is a flexible target that should be adaptable to your unique needs. For example, let's say you feel best starting to eat at a 2 on the Hunger Scale and that is where you put your star. You are meeting a friend for lunch, and you do a mindful pause for hunger before ordering and notice that you are just starting to feel mild hunger, around a 1 on the scale. Do you skip lunch, sipping on water while you watch your friend eat, only to walk out of the restaurant, reach your preferred 2 on the scale, and get a sandwich at the corner deli? No, hopefully we can use the Hunger Scale flexibly and practically. In this situation, for most of us, that would mean having lunch with your friend, even if it means starting to eat at an earlier point on the Hunger Scale than is ideal.

Wherever on the scale you decide to start eating, it is important that (as much as possible) you have food available so you can satisfy your hunger. Eating when you are hungry is part of reestablishing (or establishing for the first time) a trusting relationship with your body. It helps you develop a relationship of mutuality where you can listen to what your body is asking for and meet its needs as best as you can; in return, your body cares for you as best as possible. As you start to recognize your body's innate signs of hunger, you may notice that hunger strikes at unpredictable and inconvenient times. *I'm hungry at 10 a.m.? I still have two hours until my lunch break! I'm about to start a meeting!* You may realize that the times you have set aside in your daily schedule to eat don't align with your body's natural hunger rhythms. You may even notice variability in your hunger day-to-day.

As you get to know your hunger, over time things will likely become more consistent and predictable—or you'll just get used to the unpredictability! Especially at this early stage, I recommend you keep a stash of food handy. If you carry a purse, backpack, briefcase, satchel, or something similar, this is a great place to store some snacks. Your car or jacket pockets can also serve this purpose. If you spend a lot of time in an office, keep some snacks at work too. The idea is to have food with you so that you can satisfy hunger that may unexpectedly arise. I like foods that are shelf-stable so that if I don't eat it, I don't have to worry about it going bad. Items like granola or energy bars, nuts, dried fruit, chocolates or other candies, maybe an apple or banana (although I run the risk of finding it weeks later, brown and mushy at the bottom of my bag). I just leave my snacks in my purse until I eat them. If you are the kind of person who will remember to replace your snacks each evening, more power to you. Feel free to include stuff that needs some level of refrigeration (but ideally that can last at room temperature during the time you are out of the house). Parents who are already schlepping around snacks for your kids, make sure you have your own snacks in there too!

These foods may not always be exactly what you are in the mood to eat, but they can address your hunger until you can get to something more satisfying. They are practical and generally enjoyable choices that you can eat quickly; if, for example, you are stuck in a long meeting and start to feel hungry, you can step outside under the guise of using the restroom and eat something to satisfy your hunger. You know your lifestyle best, so the specifics will vary based on your unique needs, but the main takeaway point is to make sure that you have food available at all times of the day.

Worried you'll eat all your snacks at once? If you have a history of eating in ways that feel out of control or of binge eating, it can feel scary to always have food available. You may have been taught that the solution to controlling your eating is to limit your availability to food. This new approach can feel daunting and uncomfortable. Initially you may feel haunted by the food, like your snacks are calling for you to eat them from the recesses of your desk drawer or purse. If you want to eat the food, eat the food. But eat it mindfully, with compassion and without judgment. The intention of this practice is *not* to see how long you can keep a container of nuts in your bag without eating it. If you eat more than feels comfortable, respond to your body with kindness. What do you need in that moment? If you get a bellyache, would a heating pad or some mint tea help ease your discomfort? If you feel tired, can you rest for a bit? If you notice your inner critic acting up, try to label those thoughts, ground yourself in the present moment by focusing on your breath, and recognize that your thoughts are not your truth (for a refresher on coping with your inner critic, you can return to chapter 4). Most importantly, don't allow this experience to shake your trust in yourself. If you eat all your snacks at once, this doesn't mean that you can't be trusted around snacks, that you shouldn't keep these foods around, or that you should restrict or limit your access in any way. Quite the opposite, this means that you are still recalibrating after periods of restrictive eating and diet mentality and that you should continue giving yourself unrestricted access to food. Over time, with continued and regular access to food, we start to trust that food is always available to us, and we feel less compelled to eat it all at once. Your body will regulate. If you eat all your snacks, be sure to replenish and restock and continue forward on your path to food freedom.

Food availability can be hampered by financial constraints. If you don't have an unlimited snack budget, or if you aren't sure where your next meal is coming from, it is difficult to feel secure that food will always be available to you whenever you want it. Food insecurity can make it hard to honor your hunger and fullness cues as well as make choices about what to eat. I wish I had a nugget of wisdom to offer to solve this issue; unfortunately, all I can do is validate that this is a difficult situation that makes mindful eating more challenging—but not impossible. At its essence, mindful eating is simply the act of being present with your body and your eating experiences, whatever may arise. As is true with everything in this book, the practices are invitations that you can adapt to best meet your unique needs with compassion and acceptance.

Michael was hesitant to reconnect with his hunger. He felt virtuous subsisting on as little food as possible and worried that eating more would make him gain weight. He didn't want to return to living in a stigmatized body, especially not after he had gotten a taste of what it was like to navigate the world in a thinner body and all the privileges that afforded him. "What do you think will happen to my body if I listen to my hunger? Will I eat more? Will I gain weight?" He looked to me for reassurance, to say "don't worry, you won't gain weight. I won't let you get fat again." But I couldn't do that. I didn't know what would happen to his body if he started eating mindfully. He may gain weight, he may lose weight, he may stay the same. I didn't have a crystal ball and had no way of forecasting the future. What I did know, though, was that what Michael was doing now wasn't working for him. He was fighting against his body and holding on by a thread. And that thread was starting to fray.

As Michael learned about the strong biological mechanisms he was fighting against and how ignoring his hunger contributed to him feeling out of control with food at night, he decided to take a leap of faith and start feeding his hunger. He cut back on the supersized coffees and started to eat breakfast. He played with eating at different levels of hunger and, initially, felt most comfortable starting to eat around a 1 or 2 on the Hunger Scale. After so many years of ignoring his hunger, he liked knowing that he could eat as soon as his hunger sensations emerged. He also worried that he would feel out of control again if he got too hungry. Michael was surprised that it didn't take as much food as he would've thought to satisfy his hunger; but it felt like he was eating all the time. With these smaller meals and snacks his hunger returned frequently throughout the day. He kept snacks with him, but it was burdensome to step outside the classroom to eat something quickly several times a day when he was teaching. He continued to experiment with eating at different points on the scale and eventually settled at a 2 or 3, when he had an appetite for a more substantial meal that could keep him satiated through his teaching sessions.

As Michael started to feel more secure that his hunger needs would be cared for, his relationship with food became more playful. He experimented with different types of foods, becoming, for the first time in his life, an adventurous eater. On the weekends, he would travel to different neighborhoods in the city, seeing the sights and trying the local delicacies. Deli from the East Village, Chinese food in Flushing, Italian on Arthur Avenue; he explored places he had never been to before and ate delicious foods that he previously shunned. His life expanded beyond the confines of his studio apartment. Ironically, by allowing himself to enjoy food again and consistently satisfy his hunger, Michael became less fixated on food. He wasn't constantly thinking about what to eat and what not to eat. His hunger signals became second nature as, almost instinctively, he sensed when he was hungry, ate, and then, incredibly, went on with his day.

TAKE-ACTION ACTIVITIES

Keep meditating!

Continue to meditate for five minutes daily, using either the guided meditation available at www.drconason.com/diet-free-revolution/ or a timer, and lead yourself through the mindfulness of breath practice with the instructions in chapter 3. If you are struggling to practice consistently, revisit the strategies outlined in chapter 3 about setting up a meditation practice. If the place, time of day, or anything else isn't working for you, change it up and see if you can find something that works better.

Explore by journaling

Answer the following questions in your journal:

- What are your associations with hunger?
  - Is it "good" or "virtuous" to be hungry?
  - Do you see hunger as something to be fought against or ignored?
  - Are you scared to experience hunger?
- Do you trust that you will be able to satisfy your hunger when it arises?
- What emotions arise in connection to feeling hungry?

Understand your hunger better

Complete the blank Hunger Scale available at www.drconason.com/diet -free-revolution/ with the physical symptoms that you experience when you feel hungry. You can use the sample scale for guidance, but remember that your hunger symptoms may be different from the sample ones. It is important to focus on what your unique body is telling you. There is no one "right" answer.

If you are having difficulty identifying hunger, experiment with delaying eating and see if you can watch your hunger emerge. Note the sensations that you experience as you move through the points on the scale. No need to let yourself get so hungry that you feel sick! Eat at a comfortable level of hunger, and make sure you have food available to satisfy your hunger when the time is right.

Practice the mindful pause for hunger before, during, and after eating, as well as periodically throughout the day. If you set a random interval timer to remind you to take mindful pauses throughout the day, expand your awareness to include your hunger when the timer rings. You will continue this practice for the duration of this program until it becomes second nature and automatic. If you would like to listen to a guided audio version of the mindful pause for hunger, you can find that at www.drconason.com/diet-free-revolution/.

Eat a mindful meal focusing on awareness of hunger. Do a mindful pause for hunger prior to eating and identify your level of hunger. As you eat, pay close attention to how your hunger changes. For example, if you start eating at a 3 on the Hunger Scale, can you sense when your hunger decreases to a 2? Can you sense when it goes down to a 1? Can you detect the moment when you no longer feel hungry, when your hunger has been satisfied?

Pack your snack stash and keep it well stocked. When you eat something from your stash, replenish.

Scan your whole body for cues

Practice the body scan meditation using the instructions in the guided audio recording available at www.drconason.com/diet-free-revolution/. This meditation helps increase awareness of your body's physical cues and sensations. For this practice, you will assume a comfortable seated or lying down position and direct your attention to each part of your body, starting with the tips of your toes and moving upward along your body, all the way to the top of your head, noticing all the sensations that are present.

6

STEP 6: Finding Fullness

Tracy's life was a constant battle against her hunger and fullness. After decades of dieting, she was never sure if she would be able to satisfy her hunger when it called to her. Growing up, Tracy ate precisely measured dietetic meals that were rarely satisfying. It felt shameful to acknowledge her hunger, a reminder of the insatiable appetite she believed made her body so unruly. As a child Tracy was often kept up at night by her growling stomach and hunger pangs. It was only when she took matters into her own hands, away from her mother's watchful eye, that she was able to satisfy her hunger with secretive late-night binge episodes. When Tracy was old enough to go out on her own, she found more opportunities to fill herself. After school she would stop at the deli down the block and buy packaged pastries, chips, and candy—foods that her mother would never let her have—and eat it all on her walk home, throwing out the wrappers in the neighbor's trash, which they conveniently kept at the bottom of their driveway, to hide the evidence. When she was invited for dinner at a friend's house, she would have two or three helpings, filling her belly to the brim. She was in awe of how parents of her friends—especially her best friend, Carol, who was also chubby—allowed them to eat as much as they wanted. At Carol's house, meals were served family style and there was always more than enough to go around. Everyone ate the same thing—no special diet meals for the fat members of the family. Carol's mom commended Tracy on what a good eater she was, taking pride that Tracy enjoyed the food she cooked. "You really like that pot roast! I added some cola in the sauce, shhh, it's a secret," she would mock-whisper to Tracy over the dinner table. There was no shame around food at Carol's house, and Tracy always went to bed full. Tracy tried to spend as much time as possible at Carol's, not just because she was well-fed but because it was a rare space where her body wasn't seen as a problem.

Fullness reminded Tracy that she had autonomy over her eating. She could do what she wanted and eat what she wanted. Fullness was her rebellion. She wasn't going to be the good girl; she wasn't going to follow the rules. It was a silent rejection of the confines her mother enacted on her. As an adult, Tracy rebelled against the systems of oppression she had internalized. Although her mother had died ten years prior, she still heard her voice. Only now, it came from within: *get control of yourself, you should be ashamed of yourself for eating like that, that's not how a lady eats.* It wasn't just her mother's voice (it never was)—it was her doctor who told her to lose weight, the clothing companies that didn't make her size, the characters on television who never looked anything like her (unless they were the villain or the butt of the joke), the nasty looks from strangers when she sat next to them on the subway, the skinny moms who talked about how fat they were, the war on "obesity," the incessant hatred for her body that she faced at every turn. When she binged, she said "eff you" to all of it. Binging was *her* moment to capture, one of the few in her life not dedicated to caring for someone else, doing what other people demanded of her, or performing the role that others expected.

Tracy cherished her fullness. "It's like I'm being hugged from the inside," she described to the group. "A warm feeling rushes over me, like my own body is embracing me." With her history of chronic dieting and restrictive mindset around food, it was hard for Tracy to feel secure that food would be available to her when she needed it.

"I eat preemptively," she explained. "I'm worried that I'll get hungry and won't be able to eat, so I just eat whenever I have the opportunity, as long as I'm not totally stuffed." It was challenging for Tracy to allow herself to vacillate between states of hunger and fullness, so instead she went between feeling slightly full and completely stuffed, doing her best to avoid hunger. While some fullness was comforting, too much fullness was painful. Sometimes she would get so full that she felt sick. She would eat until she didn't have a millimeter of empty space left in her stomach and it felt like she physically couldn't manage one more bite.

In the first few weeks of the program, Tracy did a lot of work establishing a trusting relationship with her body. As we learned in chapter 5, this involved consistently feeding her body when she felt hungry and making sure she always had snacks with her. It also involved working through her restrictive mindset around food, so she could feel secure that she could eat what she wanted when she wanted it. Feeling confident that food was always available lessened her fear of hunger. She discovered that eating was more enjoyable when she felt moderately hungry (around a 2 on the Hunger Scale), and she started to welcome the early experiences of hunger because she knew they meant delicious and satisfying eating experiences were around the corner. In individual therapy, she processed her painful childhood experiences of hunger and was able to develop compassion for herself as a child. She didn't always get the parenting that she needed as a child, but now as an adult she could become her own loving caregiver. From this place of self-care and compassion, Tracy was able to tune in to her hunger and fullness in new ways.

Prior to joining the group, it was hard for Tracy to stop eating when she was comfortably full. Each meal felt like her last chance to eat. If she was enjoying something delicious, she had to eat it all now because she wasn't sure when she would be able to eat it again. Living in New York City and being financially stable, even comfortable, Tracy had pretty much any food available to her morning, noon, or night. Whether she wanted authentic Shanghai soup dumplings, pizza, or a famous New York bagel and schmear, it's never more than a few taps away. When Tracy was able to trust that she could always have access to satisfying foods without restricting herself, it became easier for her to stop eating once she was at a comfortable level of fullness. In fact, she discovered that she enjoyed food the most when she was hungry, and once she reached a comfortable level of fullness, eating past that point was no longer pleasurable (in the next chapter we will talk more about how taste changes as we eat). Now when she was eating a delicious food and hit that comfortable level of fullness, she preferred to pack up the rest of her meal and save it for the next eating experience, knowing she would enjoy it more when she was hungry.

When she first started taking home scrumptious leftovers, she would sometimes feel preoccupied with the food in her fridge, as if it were calling her name. Even though she wasn't hungry, she would go back and eat it, just so she could stop thinking about it. Rather than seeing this as confirmation that she couldn't trust herself, Tracy leaned into these feelings and allowed herself to eat the food when it called to her. This was an important part of the process because it helped Tracy trust that she really could have the food whenever she wanted it. She also realized that eating the food when she was already full brought her to an uncomfortable level of fullness and that she didn't enjoy that sensation. Over time, as she became more trusting that food would always be available when she wanted it, she became less preoccupied with the food in her fridge. Sometimes she would even discover week-old leftovers from a delicious meal that had been forgotten about in the recesses of her fridge. Spoiled, the remnants would be tossed, but if she was in the mood for that meal again, she would make sure to get herself a fresh version. The security in knowing that she would always be able to eat enjoyable foods again, whenever she wanted, laid the foundation for Tracy to listen to her internal GPS and use hunger and fullness signals to guide her eating.

What Happens in Our Body When We Feel Full?

Fullness, like hunger, is an important biological process that our body uses to guide our eating. While we are eating, food fills our belly. Our stomach temporarily expands, or distends, to accommodate the bulk of incoming food (an elastic stomach! How cool is our body?). When our stomach is distended, nerves send signals from our gut to our central nervous system that stimulate satiety centers in our brain. After food passes through our stomach into the small intestine, our stomach contracts back to its non-fed state. Once in our small intestine, nutrients including glucose (remember from chapter 5, that's the brain's fuel) are absorbed through the wall of the intestine into the bloodstream. When glucose is detected, our pancreas secretes the hormones insulin and amylin. Amylin helps slow the digestive process, so we don't get a blood sugar spike, and insulin helps transport glucose from the bloodstream into the cells. These hormones also trigger satiety signals in the brain telling us that we can stop eating now. During this time, our fat cells expel leptin (the "satiety hormone"), which triggers the brain to decrease hunger-causing neuropeptide Y and stimulate appetite-suppressing neurons. It's a beautiful dance that our body does to let us know we've had enough to eat.

Our body has early-stage and later-stage signs of fullness. Stomach distention (the stretch of your stomach to accommodate the food you've eaten) is an earlier sign of fullness, and it's what we focus on in the Fullness Scale, which we'll learn about soon in this chapter. (Another early sign of fullness is change in taste, which we'll learn about in the next chapter.) The hormonal indicators of fullness come a little later in the eating process, anywhere between five and twenty minutes after food enters our belly.[1] You may have heard that it takes your body twenty minutes to register fullness—this is where that comes from. It has spawned 1,001 dieting tips about the importance of eating slowly. But if we are mindfully attuned, we can use information from different sources in our body to register fullness in real time.

Mindful Eating with Diabetes

If you have diabetes, you may be wondering if what I've described applies to you. After all, your body may not produce or detect insulin, so does it still send out the same satiety signals? Can you practice mindful eating if you have diabetes? For most people with diabetes, hunger and fullness respond similarly to what I've described. In a randomized controlled trial of adults with type 2 diabetes, researchers found that a three-month mindful eating program was associated with significant improvements in both eating behaviors and diabetes control.[2]

With diabetes, it is important to work with your physician to come up with a treatment plan that works for you. In some cases, diabetes that is not adequately controlled can cause increased hunger (from lack of glucose absorption) or increased fullness (from delayed gastric emptying). If possible, seek out a weight-inclusive or Health at Every Size–informed endocrinologist. You may remember from chapter 2 that fat people are subject to subpar medical care. Type 2 diabetes (also called insulin-resistant diabetes) is a common example of medical discrimination in action. If you are fat and develop diabetes—or even elevated blood sugar classified as "prediabetes," a condition deemed a precursor to diabetes even though fewer than 2 percent of cases progress to diabetes each year—you will most likely be given the pre-scription of weight loss.[3] Your doctor may recommend a strict diet and warn you that you will need to take medications if you can't get your diabetes under control with dietary changes—as if this is your moral imperative. Often people are given little to no guidance on how to make these changes, other than perhaps some vague edict to eliminate sugar, carbs, "white foods," fruits, certain vegetables, and more. This diet is not sustainable for most people, especially when uncontrolled diabetes is making your appetite feel out of whack. You deserve to be treated with evidence-based care, including medications that happen to be plentiful and effective for diabetes management. I've seen too many people struggle to follow a strict diet, experience deep shame when they can't maintain the diet or when binge-eating symptoms emerge, and blame themselves for their diabetes. This is especially ironic given the role that internalized weight stigma plays in type 2 dia-betes and metabolic syndrome (see chapter 2 for a refresher).

A prescription for weight loss is not evidence-based care, because there is a lack of long-term studies showing it to be feasible for most people. A recommendation to follow a strict diet that is not sustainable long-term for most people is also not evidence-based care. Each one of us has a unique body with unique needs. Discovering how your body signals hunger and fullness is a process of exploration. Whether or not you have diabetes or another metabolic condition, I encourage you to tune in and listen to what your body is telling you and how it responds to being fed.

The Fullness Scale

The Fullness Scale is a counterpart to the Hunger Scale that we learned about in the last chapter. You can find a completed version of the Fullness Scale on the next page, which includes commonly experienced sensations of fullness. It's not meant to be a universal description; that's why I encourage you to go to www.drconason.com/diet-free-revolution/, download the blank scale, and complete it with the symptoms of fullness that *you* experience.

Fullness exists on a spectrum ranging from the subtlest mild sensations to ones nearly impossible to ignore. A 0 on the Fullness Scale indicates the absence of fullness; you may feel satisfied (neither hungry nor full) or you may feel hungry. Remember that hunger and fullness are assessed separately. As you eat, if you are paying close attention, you might notice the earliest signs of fullness emerge, "slightly full" or a 1 on the Fullness Scale. Signs may include the gentle stretch or distention of our stomach. It's a whisper of fullness; if you aren't listening carefully, it is easy to miss these sensations because they are subtle.

If we continue eating, we will reach "moderately full," designated by a 2 on the Fullness Scale. This point is characterized by more moderate sensations of stretch or distention in our stomach. Our belly feels comfortable, but the fullness is more notable now, and you may also have decreased desire to eat as the satiety centers in our brain get activated. If a 1 was our stomach whispering to us, a 2 is our stomach talking to us in a clearly audible conversational voice.

If we continue eating, we will reach "very full" or a 3 on the Fullness Scale. Here we may experience significant stomach distention that may feel uncomfortable. Our pants may feel tight, we may feel tired after eating, and it may even feel a little difficult to breathe deeply as our expanded full belly creates resistance on our diaphragm. Don't worry—your lung capacity will return to normal after fullness subsides! Our body is talking to us loudly here (imagine a friend trying to get your attention in a noisy party, raising their voice to be heard above the loud music), and fullness is difficult to ignore. Some people experience discomfort at this level of fullness.

FULLNESS SCALE

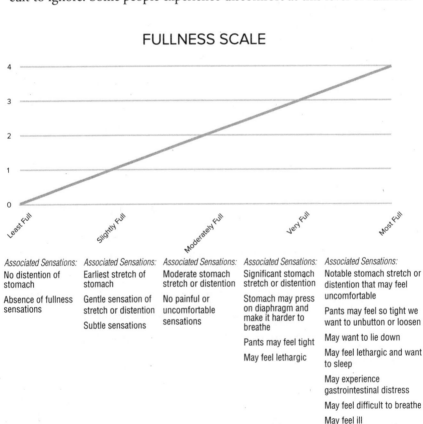

Associated Sensations:	*Associated Sensations:*	*Associated Sensations:*	*Associated Sensations:*	*Associated Sensations:*
No distention of stomach	Earliest stretch of stomach	Moderate stomach stretch or distention	Significant stomach stretch or distention	Notable stomach stretch or distention that may feel uncomfortable
Absence of fullness sensations	Gentle sensation of stretch or distention	No painful or uncomfortable sensations	Stomach may press on diaphragm and make it harder to breathe	Pants may feel so tight we want to unbutton or loosen
	Subtle sensations		Pants may feel tight	May want to lie down
			May feel lethargic	May feel lethargic and want to sleep
				May experience gastrointestinal distress
				May feel difficult to breathe
				May feel ill

If we continue eating, we will reach "most full" or a 4 on the Fullness Scale. This is when we may feel like *I'm so stuffed, I can't eat one more bite*, and there is no room left in our stomach. Our belly is notably distended now and may make clothes feel so tight that we need to unbutton our pants or lie down to relieve some pressure. We may experience gastrointestinal distress including nausea, a stomachache, or acid reflux. We may have more notable feelings of tightness in our stomach and can experience shortness of breath as our full belly restricts the movement of our diaphragm and lowers lung capacity. We may feel sleepy after eating and want to take a nap. Here our body is screaming for our attention because if we continue eating past this level of fullness, we could become ill.

Just as we learned to eat in accordance with our hunger cues in the last chapter, it is also important that we allow ourselves to eat to a comfortable level of fullness. Oftentimes we decide how much we are going to eat before we even start eating. This can range from always eating everything on your plate (the "clean plate club") to deciding that you can only eat one cookie or half your dinner serving because that is all you think is acceptable to eat. Sometimes we stop eating just because our dining companion proclaims "I'm so full" even if we are not. These external cues and rules do not take our physiological needs into account and are premised on discounting our body's internal signals. Eating in accordance with our fullness cues is another way of developing a trusting relationship with our body, where we can feel secure that we will eat as much as our body needs to feel comfortably full and always give ourselves more food when we next need it.

At what level of fullness should I stop eating? At this point in our journey together, you probably won't be surprised that there is no one universal answer. Finding the "right" level of fullness is something I invite you to explore, using the tools provided here. It's a process of getting to know your body and how to meet your unique needs. Just as most people feel uncomfortable at the upper end of the Hunger Scale, the upper end of fullness can bring discomfort as well. As we familiarize ourselves with fullness and experiment with where the most comfortable place is to stop eating, we won't always get it "right." There will be times that we walk away from a meal and then feel hungry soon after, realizing we didn't eat quite enough. Make sure that you always have food available to you, so you can simply go back and eat some more. We will also have times that we leave a meal and feel uncomfortably full. Eating past comfortable fullness is something almost everyone experiences at one time or another. It is a normal part of the human experience. If you eat past the point of comfortable fullness, tend to yourself with compassion. What do you need most at this moment? How can you help your body feel better? If you have a bellyache, would some warm mint tea help soothe it? Would changing into looser clothes be more comfortable? If you feel sleepy from overeating, can you take a nap? Or perhaps a slow walk is what you need?

Sometimes it can be tough to stop eating when we've had enough to eat. This can happen for a number of reasons. For starters, when we are really enjoying our meal, we don't want that pleasurable experience to end. It's hard to say goodbye, or even "see you later," to delicious food. As we'll learn in the next chapter, tuning in to taste (which changes as we get full) can help us decipher if we are still deriving pleasure from the food. Trusting that you can always have this food again whenever you want can help ease the goodbye. It's also okay to feel sad when your eating experience comes to an end. If we've been looking forward to a meal, there can be disappointment when the experience has ended. If the meal was a rare moment of pleasure in your day, you can feel down when your "reward" is over. Sometimes the ending of a meal brings up unresolved feelings of grief and loss. If we're using food to disconnect from or numb difficult emotions, we may feel despondent when that tool has run its course. We can allow those feelings to be there without doing anything to force them away (more on coping with uncomfortable feelings and emotional eating in chapter 9).

Overeating (defined here as eating past the point of comfortable fullness) can bring out our harsh inner critic, internalizations of the fatphobic messages we receive from our culture. Despite the fact that weight is overwhelmingly determined by genetics (studies suggest that genes account for as much as 80 percent of the variance in our weight), diet culture attributes fatness to overeating.[4] As we learned in chapter 2, most people—including health care professionals—believe that people are fat because they eat too much. Hence, fatness becomes synonymous with overeating and is associated with negative individual attributes like gluttony, lack of control, lack of discipline, and laziness. When we overeat, we feel shame around our body and berate ourselves for not being more disciplined. In puritanical fashion, "overindulging" is a mortal sin. In the 1995 horror film *SE7EN*, a serial killer targets people he believes are guilty of one of the seven deadly sins. Gluttony is represented by a fat person who the killer forces to literally eat himself to death. If you've ever seen the movie, it's a scene that stays with you, perhaps because the killer's hatred of fat people is both terrifying and commonplace. In our culture few things are as villainized as much as fat people eating. If a fat person dares to post a picture of themselves eating on social media, they will commonly be met with dehumanizing insults and violent threats. People in larger bodies are often harassed while eating at restaurants or shopping at a grocery store. When you notice your inner critic berating you for having eaten past comfortable fullness, try to recognize where this voice comes from and what systems profit off your believing these lies. When you sense your inner critic berating you for overeating, simply notice this voice, label it, and ask yourself how you can best care for yourself with compassion in this moment.

Mindful Pause for Fullness

Let's integrate fullness into our mindful pause exercises. To take a mindful pause to check in with fullness, do the following:

1. Get into your meditative position with a dignified upright posture and your feet flat on the ground, or whatever posture your body is calling for at the moment.

2. Bring your full awareness to your breath for three or four breath cycles.

3. Expand your awareness to focus on your belly. Do you notice any sensations of fullness? Think about the Fullness Scale (where 0 is

the absence of fullness and 4 is most full) and give yourself a rating. How full are you right now? How do you know that? What sensations do you notice that inform your decision?

You may sense a pull to use external factors to inform your decision of fullness. For example, you may think, *I just finished my lunch, so I must be full.* Or *it's been hours since I last ate, I couldn't possibly feel full.* Remember that these external cues are not as reliable as the internal cues our body sends us. Try your best to prioritize and trust the information from your body.

Familiarizing yourself with your hunger and fullness should be a gentle and curious exploration of how to compassionately care for yourself. This is not the eat-only-when-you-are-hungry-and-stop-as-soon-as-you-are-full diet. Diets don't work, remember? If you try to turn this program into a diet, it will backfire. There is no right or wrong in mindful eating, only opportunities to learn more about yourself and practice self-compassion. You can always choose to eat until you are stuffed. You can choose to eat when you are not hungry. You can choose to eat while zoning out in front of the TV. You can choose to binge. I just ask that you make those choices with kindness toward yourself. When you notice your harsh inner critic saying *you are full now, you have to stop eating,* or *you can't eat that, you aren't even hungry,* politely tell that voice to screw off, and remember that you have the autonomy to make your own decisions based on what you want to do in any given moment.

TAKE-ACTION ACTIVITIES

Meditate a bit longer

If you have consistently been meditating for five minutes daily (or most days), try increasing your meditation practice to ten or fifteen minutes daily. You can either set a timer and practice independently—walking yourself through the process of focusing on your breath, noticing when your mind wanders off, and gently bringing your awareness back to your breath—or listen to the fifteen-minute guided meditation available at www.drconason.com/diet-free-revolution/. If you would like, you are also welcome to experiment with the many different mindfulness meditations available online and through different apps (just make sure that you are doing *mindfulness* meditation; there are different types of meditation, and not all foster the same skills we are building in this program). If you have not been consistently practicing five minutes of meditation daily, stay with the five-minute time period and revisit the information provided in chapter 3 about developing a meditation practice. You may want to experiment with decreasing the time to three minutes (you can find a three-minute guided meditation at www.drconason.com/diet-free-revolution/) and see if you are better able to integrate the shorter practice period into your daily routine. Whether you are meditating for three, five, ten, or fifteen minutes, continue to meditate every day.

Explore fullness by writing

Answer the following questions in your journal:

- What are your associations with fullness?
  - Is it "sinful" or "gluttonous" to be full?
  - Is fullness shameful?
  - Is fullness comforting?
  - What emotions arise in connection to feeling full?

- Imagine that you are out to eat with a friend. After eating the appetizers, your friend announces, "I'm so stuffed." You don't feel full and are eagerly awaiting the arrival of your entrée. Do any feelings come up because your friend is full and you want to continue eating? How might you best care for yourself in this scenario?

- What emotions arise when you are uncomfortably full?

- Do you trust that you will be able to satisfy your fullness when it arises? This means eating enough to feel comfortably full.

- If you have difficulty stopping eating when you feel comfortably full, what are some reasons you notice? It may be useful to take some notes in the moment during meals or snacks when you notice you are comfortably full but want to continue eating. Are you feeling secure that this food will be available to you whenever you want it? Are there any judgments coming up around the food? Is the food helping you cope with uncomfortable emotions? Jot down whatever you're thinking about, or feeling, or noticing in your body.

- What are some ways that you can compassionately tend to yourself when you are uncomfortably full? Write down at least five options for self-care that you can engage in after you've eaten too much. Some examples include, but are not limited to, placing a heating pad on your belly, eating a ginger candy, drinking some herbal tea to calm your tummy, or going for a gentle walk. What helps you feel better when you are uncomfortably full?

Fill out the Fullness Scale

Complete the blank Fullness Scale available at www.drconason.com /diet-free-revolution/ with the physical symptoms that you experience when you feel full. You can use the sample Fullness Scale for guidance, but remember that your fullness symptoms may vary from the sample ones.

It is important to focus on what your unique body is telling you. There is no one "right" answer.

If you are having difficulty identifying fullness, next time you are eating mindfully watch as it emerges, and note the sensations as you move through the points on the scale until you reach a comfortable stopping point.

Use the mindful pause for fullness

Practice the mindful pause for fullness before, during, and after eating, as well as periodically throughout the day. If you set a random interval timer to remind you to take mindful pauses throughout the day, expand your awareness to include your fullness when the timer rings. You will continue this practice for the duration of this program until it becomes second nature and automatic.

If you would like to listen to a guided audio version of the mindful pause for fullness, you can find that at www.drconason.com/diet-free -revolution/. As a reminder, we integrated hunger into our mindful pause in the last chapter, so we can now check in for both hunger and fullness when we do our mindful pauses.

Notice your fullness mindfully

Eat a mindful meal focusing on awareness of fullness. Do a mindful pause for fullness prior to eating, and identify your level of fullness. As you eat, pay close attention to how your fullness changes. For example, if you start eating at a 0 on the Fullness Scale, can you sense the earliest signs of fullness starting to emerge? Can you identify the sensations of a 1 on the Fullness Scale? What about the more notable sensations of a 2 on the scale? As you progress on the Fullness Scale, notice where feels like a comfortable point to stop eating. Remember, you should always have food available to you. When we decide to stop eating, we must feel secure that we can always eat again next time the urge strikes.

Mindful eating with nuts

Practice mindful eating with nuts. To do this exercise, you'll need some nuts, either mixed or all one type. If you are allergic or if your body doesn't respond well to this food, substitute a similar dense snack. Put your nuts in a bowl or open container and have a seat. Start by taking a mindful pause: place your feet flat on the ground and your back upright in a dignified meditative posture; if this is not comfortable or accessible, take whatever position your body is calling for. You may close your eyes or leave them gently open in a soft downward gaze. Focus on your breath for three or four breath cycles, noticing the inhale and exhale of the breath. Next expand your awareness to focus on any sensations in your belly. Using the Hunger Scale, give yourself a number for how hungry you are. How do you know that? Using the Fullness Scale, give yourself a number for how full you are. How do you know that?

Now open your eyes and observe the nuts in front of you. Notice if any thoughts or feelings come up as you prepare to eat this food. Observe these thoughts and return your attention to the sensations occurring at this moment. Take one nut and notice as much as you can about its appearance, shape, color, and texture. Bring it up to your nose and smell it, noticing if there is any scent. When you are ready, place the nut in your mouth and notice as much as you can about the taste as you chew and swallow it.

After you have eaten the first nut, give yourself ratings again on the Hunger and Fullness Scales. Did your numbers change at all from before you started eating? Lead yourself through the same process of mindfully eating a second nut, noticing the appearance, smell, and taste. When you have finished eating the second nut, give yourself ratings on the scales. Have the numbers changed at all? Continue leading yourself through the process of eating the nuts mindfully, giving yourself a hunger and fullness rating after each nut, until you notice changes in your hunger and fullness and reach a point where you would like to stop eating. This exercise is also available in an audio format at www.drconason.com/diet-free-revolution/.

Tinker with portions

Experiment with different portion sizes. Now that we are tuning in to the fullness signals that our body is sending us, we will focus on prioritizing that information above external cues like how much food is on our plate. Play with intentionally putting more or less food on your plate, taking second or third or fourth helpings, and/or leaving food on your plate. For example, you may want to see what it is like to put a small portion on your plate and give yourself multiple servings until you reach a comfortable level of fullness. Or take more than you think you'll eat and plan to leave some food on your plate (feel free to take another helping or two if you didn't take enough in the first serving).

Are there emotions that arise at seeing a small amount of food on your plate, eating everything on your plate, taking multiple servings, or having food left on your plate? You can journal about any feelings that come up. As always, make sure that food is consistently available to you so that you can have enough to eat. As we eat according to our internal cues, we may start to notice that the amount of food we are served is less or more food than we want to eat. Consequently, we may find ourselves taking additional helpings or leaving food on our plate as we practice eating in accordance with our body's internal GPS.

7

STEP 7: Embrace Your Yum
Tuning In to Taste

*L*inda came into group session looking repentant. As we went around the group, checking in with how each participant was doing, Linda said: "It's been a rough week. I've been trying to eat what I want, but I really think that there are some foods I just can't keep in control of. Like chocolate. I'm a chocoholic." She laughed that nervous giggle. It only lasted for a moment until her face dropped back down into a glum frown. "I'm serious, though, maybe I just shouldn't allow myself to eat chocolate."

I asked Linda to share more about her experience. "I was in Magnolia Bakery, my absolute favorite bakery, and I always see this cake there. German chocolate. When I was dieting, I used to go in there and play a game with myself; if I was going to get a slice of cake, which one would I get? Red velvet, coconut, hummingbird ... they all looked so delicious, but the German chocolate stands out from the rest with its three layers of cake and coconut caramel frosting. Of course, I would never allow myself to get the cake. I would just get my cup of coffee and go. But now, with this program, I said screw it, I'm getting the damn cake. And I didn't just get one slice, I got two! I don't know if you've ever had their cake but it's an enormous portion. I figured I would eat half a slice when I got home and save the other slice and a half for later in the week.

"I was practically shaking as I brought the cake home. I felt giddy with excitement but also nervous about if I would be able to control myself. As soon as I got home, I opened the container, got a fork, and took a bite. I was in ecstasy. The cake was everything I dreamed it would be. The chocolate cake was spongy and moist, the caramel dense and sweet, and the coconut shreds added the perfect texture. I had another bite and another one. Before I knew it, I had eaten more than half the cake slice. That's when my inner critic started chiming in—*you took such huge bites you pig, now it's already halfway gone.* I knew I should put the cake away—after all, I had already eaten more than I intended. But was there really a point in saving less than half the slice? I mean, I had already eaten so much of it, I thought I might as well eat the rest. I went from ecstasy to anger. *I never should've gotten the cake in the first place. This program isn't for me. My body isn't trustworthy. I have no self-control.*

"I took another bite. Now I was hate-eating the cake, I just wanted to make it go away. The remaining sliver taunted me. I knew that if I didn't finish it now, I would be thinking about it all night. I ate the last few bites and then, disgusted with myself, I opened the second slice, went to the kitchen sink, picked up the dish soap, and squeezed it all over the cake. Then I threw it in the trash."

The group sat in silence for a moment. Perhaps we were mourning the delicious slice of cake sitting in Linda's trash bathed in dish soap. Tracy was the first to speak. "I used to do that too. With the dish soap. It felt like the only way I could stop eating."

Mia chimed in. "It was salt for me. I would open the shaker and dump a pile of salt over my food so I wouldn't eat anymore. Look at us, we have so little faith in our ability to stop eating."

I asked Linda, "When was the moment that you started feeling out of control with the cake?"

She thought for a moment. "I guess it was when I realized I had eaten more than half the cake. It made me feel like I had failed since I only wanted to eat half."

"Did you *want* only half or believe you *should* only eat half? That half was the acceptable portion size?" I probed her.

"I guess the latter. Since I decided before I even got the cake home that I would only eat half, it couldn't have been a decision that was attuned to my body. I guess I still have some diet thoughts about the cake. That it's a bad food and I shouldn't eat too much."

"So maybe it's not the cake that made you feel so out of control as much as your restrictive way of thinking about it," I suggested. "Did you enjoy the cake? I know you said the first bite was incredible, but what about the other bites? Was the last bite as good as the first?" I asked.

Linda chuckled. "I don't even know. I got so lost in my thoughts, I didn't really taste most of the cake."

Linda's experience is not unusual. Think about when you eat. Do you fully taste each bite of food? Most of us don't. From an evolutionary perspective, this makes a lot of sense. Taste is one of our most primitive senses. Over a billion years ago, some of the earliest cells on the planet were taste cells that could sense chemicals in the seawater around them and know what to avoid and what to ingest.[1] While our system has evolved since early life-forms, the basic premise of taste as a mechanism to guide us in what to eat and what to avoid has remained the same. Our attention is almost always captured by the first bite of food because this is life-or-death information. It is how the earliest humans knew whether a berry they picked was a rank-tasting deadly moonseed berry or a sweet-tasting nourishing blueberry. Even today, taste (and our related sense of smell) helps us detect spoiled or otherwise dangerous food. Is that milk in the fridge with a sell-by date of last week still good? Give it a whiff. Does your chicken taste off? You won't need to take more than a bite to know it's spoiled (and then we'll probably ask someone else to taste it too—not sure what that phenomenon is all about!).

When we eat foods that are safe and nourishing, our brain rewards us by releasing the feel-good hormone dopamine. These rewards are strongest when we are hungry; it's our body's way of making sure we get nutrition when we need it. Hunger affects our enjoyment of food in (at least) two ways: by making our taste perception stronger *and* by increasing the rewards that our brain sends out in response to food. One study found that people are better able to perceive the presence of sweet and salty tastes (which indicate food is safe to eat and a good source of energy) in a solution when they are hungry.[2] Their sensitivity to bitter tastes (associated with poisonous foods) was not impacted by hunger. Research suggests that these changes in taste can be attributed to a neural circuit in the hypothalamus (the appetite control center in our brain) that increases our preference for sweet foods when hungry.[3] There is a reason people say hunger is the best seasoning. As we eat and become satisfied, our taste perception becomes less sensitive and our brain's response to food becomes less rewarding. In short, the taste of food becomes less enjoyable as we eat. This is another way that our body guides our eating—but we must pay attention to use these valuable (and delicious) cues.

While our awareness is swiftly captured by the first bite of food, once we've gotten the all-clear that a food is safe to eat, our attention is free to wander. If we are not eating mindfully, we make decisions about how much to eat based on the memory of the taste of the first few bites of food combined with external cues such as how much food is on our plate or when our dining companion stops eating. You know how when you look at a star in the sky, you are seeing the star as it was thousands of years ago? That's kind of how many of us are making decisions around food. We are looking at a past moment in time (the first bites of food) as if it were the present and then making decisions about how much to eat based on outdated information from an earlier time. Worst of all, we are missing the enjoyment of the eating experience!

As legendary chef Julia Child said, "We should enjoy food and have fun. It is one of the simplest and nicest pleasures in life."[4] Mindfulness can help us connect with the pleasure in food (and life). Diet culture robs us of seeking pleasure in food; we are indoctrinated into the "food is fuel" mentality and believe that if we give in to the hedonic pleasures of eating, we have succumbed to our animalistic desires. It shames us for experiencing bodily pleasures, leading us to eat with conflict and disconnection. What would it be like to rebel against these oppressive norms and engage in the radical act of pleasure?

Taste Enjoyment Scale

The Taste Enjoyment Scale is a tool we can use to connect with our taste and enjoyment of foods. It is a rating instrument that ranges from 0 to 10. A 0 indicates that the food is not enjoyable; you may dislike the taste of the food or have a more neutral experience, but the taste of the food is not eliciting pleasure. A 5 on the scale indicates moderate pleasure; you are enjoying the food but it's not your favorite taste. A 10 is the most pleasure you could imagine deriving from a bite of food. It's like fireworks are going off in your mouth, and you are in ecstasy from the overwhelming pleasure of the taste of the food. These are the reference points of the scale; you can use the numbers in between to fine-tune your ratings (e.g., a bite that is very enjoyable but not the absolute best thing you've ever eaten may be a 7 or 8 on the Taste Enjoyment Scale). There are no rights or wrongs here; it's just a tool to help you explore your enjoyment of the taste of foods.

Have you ever noticed that the taste of food changes as we eat? Taste, another part of our internal GPS, guides our eating by decreasing the pleasure we derive from eating as we get full. It is one of our early signs of fullness. As our stomach registers food and digestion takes place, signals are sent to our brain to inhibit the reward process. Our taste sensitivity decreases and the dopamine release in our brain slows down. Essentially

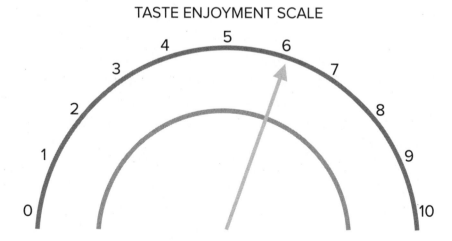

TASTE ENJOYMENT SCALE

our body is sending us signals that we've had enough to eat; we are adequately nourished and it's okay to stop eating now.

Prior to practicing mindful eating, I was never consciously aware of these changes in taste. But I did have a habit of reaching for the saltshaker midway through a meal. Even though I wasn't aware of what was happening, my brain was registering the food as less enjoyable. Because, at the time, I ate according to how much food was on my plate, not what my body was telling me, I would reflexively reach for the salt as I became full—the food was less enjoyable, and I was trying to recapture the initial taste of the food. Sadly, salt is not as good a seasoning as hunger.

It can feel sad and disappointing to realize that the food we are eating is no longer as enjoyable as it once was. Just as when we recognize that our fullness is bringing an eating experience to an end, we may feel a sense of grief and loss as taste diminishes toward the end of a meal. After all, it is human nature to want to prolong pleasurable experiences and hold on to them as long as we can. Part of mindfulness is allowing ourselves to simply experience these feelings as they arise, without needing to push them away. If you feel sad and disappointed at the loss of pleasure or want to hold on to the eating experience, wishing that it would return to its initial enjoyment (much as I did with my futile attempt to salt my food back to full flavor), simply notice these feelings. You can label them ("sadness," "emotion," "yearning," etc.) and refocus your awareness on your breath or your eating experience. I want to reiterate here that trusting we can eat enjoyable foods again whenever we want them is essential to being able to listen to our body and eat in accordance with our internal cues. Personally I really enjoy leftovers for this reason. When I'm eating a yummy meal and feel fullness setting in and the taste of the food is less pleasurable, I take comfort in knowing that I can stop eating now and save the remainder of the meal for another time when I'm hungry again and my taste buds will be reset to experience the full pleasure of the food.

At your next meal or snack, use the Taste Enjoyment Scale to tune in to your experiences with taste. Prior to eating, do a mindful pause for hunger and fullness. Sit in a meditative position with your feet flat on the floor and your spine in an upright posture, or whatever posture your body is calling for. You can close your eyes if you would like or leave them open with a soft gaze toward the floor in front of you. Focus on your breathing for three or four breath cycles, noticing the breath as it enters and exits your body. Then expand your awareness to focus on your stomach. How hungry are you? Using the Hunger Scale, give yourself a rating from 0 to 4, where 0 is not hungry and 4 is most hungry. How full are you? Using the Fullness Scale, give yourself a rating between 0 and 4, where 0 is least full and 4 is most full. Open your eyes and take a moment to look at the food in front of you. Then bring the food up to your nose and smell it. When you are ready, put a bite of the food in your mouth. Hold it in your mouth without biting it and give the food a rating using the Taste Enjoyment Scale. From 0 to 10, how much do you enjoy the taste of the food? Now bite into the food and see if the taste changes. Give yourself another rating on the Taste Enjoyment Scale. When you have finished chewing and swallowing the first bite, take another bite of food and give yourself another rating on the Taste Enjoyment Scale. Continue eating, giving yourself a rating on the Taste Enjoyment Scale with each bite. Check in with your hunger and fullness as well. Continue eating until you feel satisfied or choose to stop eating. Did you notice any changes in the taste of food as you ate?

Smell plays a role in our taste of foods. Humans have a short passage that runs from our mouth to our nasal cavity, which allows us to sense the aromatic component of flavor as food is chewed.[5] So we are actually smelling our food with our mouth! Pretty incredible, right? If you ever want to see how integral smell is to our sense of taste, try holding your nose closed and eating something. Then release your nose and see if the taste changes. There is usually a notable difference. If you have ever suffered a bad head cold, you may not even need to do this experiment since you know firsthand how a stuffy nose affects your sense of taste. Mouth smelling is most active when we exhale and food volatiles are transported through the passage from our mouth to our nasal cavity. This is why wine connoisseurs sometimes take a sip of wine and then purse their lips and suck in air through their mouth and exhale through their nose to maximize the taste of the wine. Next time you eat, try holding the food in your mouth for a moment, taking a deep breath in through your mouth, and then exhale through your nose (careful not to choke!), and see if the flavor of the food changes at all.

Our tongue tastes the flavors sweet, salty, sour, bitter, and umami (a savory taste characteristic of meat, broths, mushrooms, and fermented products like miso, soy sauce, and cheese). There is ongoing debate about if we have specific receptors that detect the taste of fat. You may have learned about the "tongue map," a favorite diagram in elementary school classrooms that shows how certain parts of the tongue detect certain flavors. It is often depicted with the sweet taste receptors on the front of the tongue, salty and sour on the sides of the tongue, umami in the middle, and bitter all the way in the back. The tongue map was debunked in a 2006 study published in *Nature* that found we can taste all the flavors throughout our tongue, as well as in our throat and the roof of our mouth.[6] But receptors may be more intense for certain flavors in specific areas of the mouth.[7] This gives us another way to observe the taste of food. Next time you eat, try to notice where in your mouth you taste the food.

In mindfulness we cultivate *shoshin*, or "beginner's mind." It is the practice of approaching an experience as if it were your first time. Think about when you try a new food. You don't know what to expect. Because you have no memories of the food, you don't have any preconceptions of what the experience is going to be like, what the food will taste like, or if you will like it or not. We approach with curiosity and are open to possibilities. My dad used to tell a story about one of his earliest memories as a child—the first time he had ice cream. He grew up in Brooklyn, New York, and in the 1930s ice cream was a special treat (it wasn't sold in grocery stores at that time). My grandmother took him to the soda fountain to have his first ice cream. Not knowing what to expect, my dad tasted it and spit it out, exclaiming, "It's cold!" Having no prior references for this food, he assumed it was supposed to be served hot and was shocked to try the cold confection. Eventually my dad came to enjoy ice cream—strawberry was his favorite— although he rarely allowed himself to have it, because of dieting.

Similarly, memories can cloud our perception of current taste experiences. I once met a wine salesman who told me about a loyal customer who asked him to source a bottle of 1992 Montepulciano from Tuscany. The customer had enjoyed a bottle ten years before on his Italian honeymoon. He described how he and his new groom had dined alfresco overlooking the Tuscan countryside, eating panzanella and sharing this wine that tasted of boysenberry and anise, with hints of pepper and plums. He wanted to give the bottle to his husband for their ten-year wedding anniversary. After much work, the salesman was able to track down the wine and import it for his customer. The next time the customer came in, the salesman eagerly asked how the wine was. "It was terrible," the customer said. "Nothing like I remembered it, it almost tasted rancid." The wine wasn't spoiled, but it didn't meet the expectations of his glorified memory. Drinking the wine with his husband in their living room, exhausted after a long day's work, while their three children slept in the next room, just wasn't the same experience as exchanging blissful gazes in the Tuscan hills as a newlywed.

I encourage you to approach each eating experience anew, with a beginner's mind. It's not just a hypothetical exercise—because, in fact, each time we eat *is* a new experience. We have never before eaten this specific food in this exact moment in time. Try to bring a sense of wonder and exploration to your eating experiences. What will this food taste like? Will I like it? How much do I want to eat? Leave behind expectations of what you think the food will taste like, your memories of past experiences with this food, and any preconceptions you may carry. Our sense of taste is always evolving. The way we perceive flavors at one moment in time may be totally different from how we perceive them at another moment in time. With beginner's mind, we can open ourselves up to be fully present with our food and our body exactly as they are in this moment.

Food Preferences

Humans are creatures of habit and tend to prefer flavors that are familiar. For many of us, new foods can be off-putting at first, but the more that we are exposed to them, the more we start to enjoy them. For children this is especially true—they may need to be offered a new food up to twelve times before they accept it.[8] Research suggests that preferences for familiar foods start to develop even before birth as the fetus is exposed to different flavors in the amniotic fluid. In one study, infants whose mothers regularly drank carrot juice during pregnancy and breastfeeding later preferred carrot-flavored cereal.[9]

Early humans relied on this preference for familiar foods because it meant that food was likely to be safe (since it had been eaten before and hadn't killed them or made them sick). In contrast, new foods had to be approached with caution and tasted guardedly, often in small quantities, multiple times with no ill effects before they could deem these foods safe to eat with abandon. Infants and children have a higher concentration of sweet-taste receptor taste buds and are primed to prefer sweet flavors (the taste associated with safe foods) and dislike bitter ones (the taste associated with poisonous foods). This helped tykes survive because they are more likely to randomly put things in their mouths and need stronger signals to indicate which foods are safe or poisonous.

For similar evolutionary reasons, when a food (or drink) has made us sick, we develop strong aversions to that food. As a teenager I had a nasty run-in with a bottle of sake. To this day the mere smell of the alcohol makes me gag. Even eating a food around the same time as getting sick is enough to develop a lifelong dislike for the food, even if it's not what actually made us sick. For this reason, people undergoing chemotherapy are encouraged to avoid eating their favorite foods around treatments. Food aversions can also develop from negative experiences even if we don't become ill, like being forced to sit at the table for hours until you finished all your spinach. Food intolerances, in which we feel sick after eating certain foods, can also lead to diminished preferences for that food. This doesn't always happen, though, so if you developed an intolerance to a food, especially later in life, you may still desire that food, even though it doesn't make your body feel good.

Our food preferences change over time as new foods become more familiar to us (and as some familiar foods may become associated with aversive experiences). Early humans had to adapt when they moved and had to eat new local foods, so despite the early development of food preferences, they are far from locked in stone. How many of us have the same favorite foods today as when we were five years old? While we may still enjoy a good bowl of mac and cheese from the box or frozen chicken nuggets, most of us have expanded our palates to include some new favorites that we would have turned our nose up at when we were youngsters. As we get older, we can use memory and reasoning skills to determine food safety, rather than relying entirely on sweet and bland tastes. This, in combination with changes in taste perception, allows us to become more adventurous eaters. Like all the cells in our body, our taste buds die off and regenerate; taste buds die and regenerate at a rate of about every two weeks. Starting at around forty years old, when our old taste buds die off, fewer regenerate. Our sense of smell slowly starts to fade as well. This means that as we age, food tastes blander. The kimchee that tasted overwhelmingly spicy in your thirties may be a delight in your fifties. The buttered pasta that was your favorite when you were a kid needs more seasoning to be palatable as an adult. I remember ordering Sichuan Chinese food (a cuisine famous for intense spices) with my elderly grandmother and her insisting that she wanted them to add extra spice to the restaurant's spiciest dish. My eyes watered just smelling her food. She was never a fan of spicy food when she was younger, but as her sense of taste faded, she was drawn to strong flavors that she could experience.

Food preferences are another way our internal GPS guides us in what to eat. When we're looking at a menu or strolling the aisles at the grocery store, some items will look more appealing than others. For example, I love white chocolate. If I'm out to eat and see a white chocolate mousse on the menu, I will immediately be drawn to it, while I'll tend to ignore the dark chocolate desserts because they don't really float my boat (I know this is probably appalling to chocolate aficionados—I hope you don't lose faith in me!). Similarly, someone who doesn't like salty foods is likely to sail past the chip aisle at the grocery store without giving the pretzels or sour cream and onion kettle chips any thought.

While our food preferences can help guide us, they're only a piece of the puzzle. Food preferences are based on past experiences, so they're not in-the-moment data. We can hold our food preferences in mind while also being mindful of what we want to eat in the current moment. Just because a food is our favorite doesn't mean we want it right now. This is especially true when we feel secure that we can always eat this food whenever we want it. For example, let's revisit my love of white chocolate. If I'm at a restaurant and see white chocolate mousse on the menu, I may initially feel excited and want to order it. But if I check in with myself, I may discover that even though it's one of my all-time favorite desserts, I'm not really in the mood for it right now. Maybe, for whatever reason, the banana chocolate torte seems more enjoyable, even though it's not usually my go-to choice. Or maybe I'm full and don't want dessert right now. If I'm feeling like I need to get the white chocolate mousse because it's hard to find (food scarcity), perhaps I'll order one to go, so I'll know I have it when I am in the mood for it. Or I'll reassure myself that I can come back and get it when I want it. Our food preferences don't always align with what we want in the moment.

Because our preferences change over time, I like to try new foods as well as retry foods that I think I don't enjoy, bringing a beginner's mind to the experience. For example, most of my life I avoided wasabi, the spicy green mustard served alongside sushi. When I was a child, I accidentally ate it, mistaking it for avocado, and the experience was excruciating. For years I would ask sushi restaurants not to put wasabi anywhere near my meal. As a young adult, however, I tried a snack with wasabi flavoring and discovered I really liked it. Now wasabi is one of my favorite flavors and I can't imagine eating sushi without it! Mindfulness and beginner's mind can also help us assess if we are really enjoying the foods we eat regularly. When I teach mindful eating, we usually start out with mindfully eating a raisin. I can't tell you how many times people have discovered in doing this exercise that they don't like raisins, despite eating them every morning in their breakfast cereal or as a snack in trail mix. When our eating goes on autopilot, it is hard to discern what we really enjoy.

Taste Enjoyment and Digestion

Enjoying your food can help you digest better. Digestion is governed by our autonomic nervous system, the regulatory system that manages many of our unconscious bodily processes. The fact that we keep breathing, even when we are not thinking about breathing, is thanks to our autonomic nervous system. Stress is also regulated by this system; when we are in danger (or perceive ourselves to be in danger), our sympathetic nervous system (fight-or-flight response) is activated, and our body takes immediate action to keep us safe. When we are in fight-or-flight, our body prioritizes immediate lifesaving actions. As a result, non-immediate functions—like digestion and our appetite system—shut down. Think about it: if you are being chased by a lion, it's not a very opportune time for your body to signal you to stop and grab a sandwich or use the bathroom.

In fight-or-flight our body directs blood flow away from our digestive system, which can lead to constipation, diarrhea, and bloating. To give us energy to evade danger, our body also releases more glucose into the bloodstream, which can lead to insulin spikes. Unfortunately, our nervous system has a tough time differentiating real dangers, like being chased by a lion, and perceived stressors, like our inner critic berating us as we eat a bowl of ice cream. When we eat with conflict, anger, guilt, or shame, we are eating with our fight-or-flight system in action and our digestive system shut down.

In contrast, when we eat with pleasure, our parasympathetic nervous system ("rest-and-digest" response) is activated. The experience of pleasure makes us relax and signals to our body that we are safe. In a resting state, our body focuses on longer-term life-sustaining processes like digestion, along with sleep and sex (the parasympathetic nervous system is also called the "feed-and-breed" system). Blood flow is directed to your digestive tract, where the muscles are now relaxed and can release digestive juices. Saliva is stimulated in the mouth, enabling the first phase of digestion. Peristalsis (the contraction and relaxation of intestinal muscles) is enabled, which pushes food through the digestive tract and allows nutrient absorption and waste elimination.

A research study examined iron absorption in a group of Thai and Swedish participants.[10] Researchers found that when participants were given foods from their home countries (i.e., when people from Thailand were fed Thai food), which were familiar and more enjoyable, they absorbed about 50 percent more iron from the meal than when they were given foods from the other country (i.e., when people from Thailand were fed Swedish food), which were unfamiliar and less enjoyable. When the food was blended up into a mush with the same nutritional composition but sapped of any enjoyment, participants absorbed 70 percent less iron.[11] We focus a lot on the health impact of *what* we eat, but maybe we really should be focusing on how we *feel* when we eat.

Research suggests that mindful eating can increase your enjoyment of foods, therefore increasing the pleasure of your eating experiences and fostering a relaxed rest-and-digest state of the parasympathetic nervous system. In one study, participants who mindfully ate a piece of chocolate reported increased enjoyment of the chocolate compared with participants who ate the chocolate while their attention was focused on another task.[12] Interestingly, even though participants enjoyed the food more when they ate mindfully, they did not eat more, perhaps because they were also more attuned to satiation cues. In addition to enhancing the benefits of enjoying your eating experiences by seeking pleasure in the taste of your food, your daily meditation practice is also decreasing stress and allowing your body to spend more time in the parasympathetic rest-and-digest state, as it was designed to do. As we summarized in chapter 3, mindfulness is a highly effective stress-reduction technique. There are over 200 research studies showing the benefits of mindfulness, with decreased stress being one of the most robust findings.[13]

TAKE-ACTION ACTIVITIES

Maintain your meditation

Continue to meditate for three, five, ten, or fifteen minutes daily. You can either set a timer and practice independently—walking yourself through the process of focusing on your breath, noticing when your mind wanders off, and gently bringing your awareness back to your breath—or listen to the guided meditations available at www.drconason.com/diet-free-revolution/. You are also welcome to experiment with using the many guided mindfulness meditations available online or on different apps. Remember: if you are struggling to set up a consistent daily practice, you can always revisit chapter 3 for more guidance.

Be taste-aware with chocolate

Practice taste awareness with chocolate. For this exercise, you'll need some of your favorite chocolate. Get a little more than you think you would eat in one sitting. It can be a chocolate bar or truffles, milk or dark, with nuts, caramel, or nougat—anything you enjoy will work well here. If you are allergic or really dislike chocolate, feel free to substitute something similar that works better for you, like another type of candy, some cookies, or a bowl of ice cream.

Unwrap the chocolate and place it in front of you. Do a mindful pause with your feet flat on the ground and your back upright in a dignified meditative posture, or whatever position your body is calling for at this time. You may close your eyes or leave them gently open in a soft downward gaze. Focus on your breath for three or four breath cycles, noticing the inhale and exhale of the breath. Next expand your awareness to focus on any sensations in your stomach. Using the Hunger Scale, give yourself a number for how hungry you are. How do you know that? Using the Fullness Scale, give yourself a number for how full you are. How do you know that?

Now open your eyes and observe the chocolate in front of you. Notice if there are any thoughts or feelings that arise as you prepare to eat the chocolate. Observe these thoughts, and gently return your focus back to the sensations happening at this moment. Take a piece of the chocolate and notice as much as you can about its appearance, shape, color, and texture. Bring it up to your nose and smell it, inhaling the scent. When you are ready, place the chocolate in your mouth and hold it in your mouth for a moment without chewing, noticing as much as you can about the sensations that you experience. Give yourself a rating on the Taste Enjoyment Scale from 0 to 10, 0 indicating not enjoying the taste of the chocolate and 10 indicating the most delicious bite you've ever experienced. After you've given yourself a rating, move the chocolate around in your mouth or start to chew it, and give yourself another rating on the Taste Enjoyment Scale. Swallow the bite when you are ready, and notice if there are any flavors remaining in your mouth.

Pick up a second piece of chocolate and lead yourself through eating it mindfully, examining the appearance and smell, placing it in your mouth and giving yourself a rating on the Taste Enjoyment Scale, then biting into it and giving yourself another rating on the Taste Enjoyment Scale, noticing any flavors that remain in your mouth after you finish eating this piece. Did you perceive any changes in the taste of the chocolate from the first piece to the second? Continue this process of mindfully eating the chocolate focusing on the taste until you are no longer enjoying the chocolate, you feel satisfied, or you choose to stop eating. This exercise is also available in audio format at www.drconason.com/diet-free-revolution/.

Be taste-aware through a meal

Eat a mindful meal focusing on awareness of taste. Do a mindful pause for hunger and fullness prior to eating, and give yourself ratings on the Hunger and Fullness Scales. As you prepare to eat, take a moment to observe the meal with your senses, noticing the appearance, smell, and textures of the meal. When you take your first bite of food, give yourself a rating on the Taste Enjoyment Scale. As you eat, rate each bite of food on the Taste Enjoyment Scale, noticing if the taste of the food changes as you eat.

Continue using the Taste Enjoyment Scale at meals for the duration of the program, along with the Hunger Scale and the Fullness Scale. While rating your taste of food bite-by-bite is a good exercise to practice tuning in to taste, it may be more practical in your day-to-day eating to just periodically check in with yourself as you are eating to give yourself a rating on the Taste Enjoyment Scale and decide if you are still enjoying your food. Just like hunger and fullness, awareness of taste will become ingrained and automatic over time with proper practice. These exercises can be done when eating alone or with others; the ratings can be noted silently, and no one has to know that you are doing anything differently.

Be a food reviewer

Pretend you are the newest food critic for your local newspaper, and review your next meal. Don't hold back—how would you rate your meal? Five stars? Or a measly one? Describe your meal as fully as possible. What spices do you taste? Is it too salty? Would it benefit from a dash of pepper? Is the food cooked to perfection, or is it over- or undercooked? What are the textures in the food like? What do you enjoy and what could you do without?

Eat like an alien

Pretend you are an alien who has just landed on Earth from a faraway planet. You have never eaten Earth food before. At an upcoming meal or snack, try to describe your food to your alien friends back home. Remember that they have never been to this planet, so they won't understand references to other Earth foods or flavors. How can you tell them about what you're tasting? Write your description down so you can tell your alien friends all the details!

Try a new food!

Go to the market and pick out a food you've never tried before. You may want to visit a specialty store for a selection of unusual fruits and vegetables, or go to a restaurant and try a food you've never had before from a different culture. Notice any expectations that come up around eating this new food; observe and label and allow your focus to be on the taste of the new food. Observe as much as you can about the taste of this new food. Journal about the experience, describing the food in as much detail as possible.

8

STEP 8: Let Your Body Be Your Guide

How to Make Wise and Aware Choices

"Eat what I want when I want it?!" Michael, Tracy, Mia, and Linda all stared at me in disbelief. We were sailing past the midway point of the program, and all the participants were making good progress recognizing signs of hunger, fullness, and the taste of their food. But even though we had spent a lot of time talking about the hazards of dieting and disentangling health goals from weight loss, the dieting mindset continued to hang heavy in the air.

"If I eat what I want, I'll get fat again," Michael said, with a sense of panic. Clearly, his internalized weight bias was still riding strong. This was the case for most of the group; despite their emerging trust in their internal GPS to guide their eating, they were having a tough time letting go of dreams about weight loss and fears of weight gain.

"I'd just eat croissants and chocolate cake all day! I would be as big as a house," Linda stammered.

"Isn't that already what I'm doing? I obviously have no self-control," Tracy said, shame dripping from her voice.

"There is no way I can trust my body," Mia said. The rest of the group nodded in agreement.

"I know, it's scary," I said. "We are told in a thousand different ways that our body is bad, that we can't trust ourselves, and that our singular goal in life should be to devote every available resource to shrinking ourselves."

It's hard to unlearn these norms—and it's hard to live in the world in a fat body or one that society deems otherwise unacceptable. Fear of gaining weight or desire to lose weight in a fatphobic culture is to be expected. My clients commonly ask, "What will happen to my weight when I start eating mindfully? When I start eating mindfully, will I lose weight? Surely if I can stop binge eating, my weight will go down." The truth is, neither I nor anyone else has any way of predicting what will happen to your body when you stop dieting and start eating mindfully. I can tell you that one of three things will occur: your body may get smaller, your body may get larger, or your body may stay the same size. No matter what your body does, always remember that the problem is diet culture, not your body. While we can't always eliminate our internalized weight bias and body shame, we can change the way that we relate to these thoughts when they come up, as we've been practicing. Observing and labeling these thoughts about our body (as "judgment," "internalized weight bias," "cultural conditioning," "patriarchy," "oppression," or whatever label resonates with you) can help us gain distance from the thoughts and observe them without getting so lost in them. But even with this practice, trusting your body to guide your eating choices may feel like a leap of faith.

I asked the group to imagine a trapeze artist swinging between the high bars. There is a moment when the acrobat must let go of the bar they are securely swinging from and take the risk of reaching for the next bar, allowing their body to fly through space, unsure if they will make it. The first time an acrobat attempts this feat, it must be terrifying. It may even feel hard to let go of that first bar, where they are safe and stable. But if they stay on that first bar, they are stuck. They are just dangling in midair, with no way to reach the platform on the other side. So even though they aren't sure if they will make it to the next bar, they take a leap of faith. They let go of what is comfortable and move into the unknown, trusting that the path forward is better than being immobilized. Over time, after this act is practiced hundreds of times, it becomes less scary. The acrobat trusts that their body will be able to make it to the next bar. In fact, the act may even become instinctual, where their body knows how to perform the actions without consciously thinking about letting go of one bar and grasping for the next.

"Right now you are like that acrobat making the leap for the first time. You may not feel secure that you will get to the other side, but you are willing to take a leap of faith because you know that moving forward is better than being stuck flailing in midair," I concluded.

"I like that," Tracy said. "It's uncomfortable, but we can notice the discomfort and move forward anyway. We can do hard things."

"Exactly," I replied.

"But I don't even know where to start," Tracy said. "I've spent so much of my life on a diet. Eating zucchini noodles instead of pasta because that was the 'right' thing to do. Eating low-calorie frozen dessert instead of ice cream because that's what was allowed. It gave me guidance. Even though I often didn't do what I was supposed to do—or what the diet plan told me I should do—it was still how I made my decisions, how I knew if I was on track or off the rails, if I was good or bad. Without these rules, how can I trust that my body will guide me the right way?"

Does the idea of eating what you want when you want it feel scary? Do you worry that your eating will become out of control? In this chapter we will learn more about how to use our skills of identifying hunger, fullness, cravings (an urge to eat a specific food), and nonrestrictive eating (feeling secure that you are allowed to eat all foods), as well as our past experiences of how we enjoy certain foods and how they react with our body, to mindfully check in with ourselves to decide if and what we want to eat.

Diet mentality and mistrust in our body die hard. Diet culture nestles its way into the deepest recesses of our psyches and can take time to extract. It is not uncommon for people practicing mindful eating to initially hold on to judgments around food. There will likely be a time when you are coexisting with these good food/bad food thoughts (including thoughts that it's okay to eat previously restricted foods as long as you don't eat "too much," which, heads up, is also restriction and your body will respond accordingly). We'll just keep observing and labeling them (as we practiced in chapter 4) and trying to shift our awareness back to the guidance that our body is giving us, taking that leap of faith that we can listen to our body, even when we aren't quite sure if our body is trustworthy or not. Your body is here to guide and support you, whether you believe it or not.

Why Nutrition Information Isn't a Reliable Guide

There is no shortage of nutrition information available telling us what to eat and what not to eat. New "miracle superfoods" get their five minutes of fame each week. Nutrition experts tell us to eat this, not that. We are told some foods are "toxic" and others will help "detox." This guidance on which foods are "healthy" and which are "bad" changes all the time. One moment we are instructed to eat a low-fat diet and there is a run on pasta (remember the 1980s?). The next, it is revealed that carbs are bad and we all go barreling to the Atkins-sanctioned low-carb pasta brands (1990s and early aughts, I'm looking at you here). But then the "clean eating" movement comes around in the mid-2010s and tells us it's really processed food that is bad; the low-carb pasta you are eating is basically poison—how many ingredients can you pronounce on the back of the label?! So off we go, back to the pasta aisle, now seeking out a brand made with organic hand-ground artisanal flour. This happens time and time again with nutrition advice. What is healthy one minute is toxic the next.

Here are a few other examples. For decades we were told to avoid eggs (or at least egg yolks) because they cause high cholesterol. I went through years of eating egg-white omelets because I thought they were "healthy." Lo and behold, this myth has been debunked, and it is now believed that foods that *have* cholesterol in them do not *cause* high cholesterol in our body.[1] Furthermore, the yolk contains important nutrients, so it is now recommended that you include yolks in your omelet if you want to eat "healthy." Will this change again? Probably. If you search "are eggs healthy" online, you'll get a lot of different opinions, which speaks to how utterly unreliable expert advice on nutrition can be. Dairy recommendations are another example of how fickle nutrition advice is. I grew up drinking skim milk and eating fat-free yogurt because these were the recommended options. I still remember my mom adding pink packets of Sweet'N Low to her fat-free yogurt. This was considered healthy. Now that diet culture has shifted its focus away from fat and toward sugar and processed foods, full-fat dairy is seen as the healthy option—and artificial sugars like saccharin, the main ingredient in Sweet'N Low, are generally frowned upon.

Nutrition advice is often subjective, with experts picking studies that support one perspective while ignoring others. Nutrition recommendations are also heavily influenced by the financial interests of the food industry. In 2020, the scientific advisory panel convened to recommend revisions to the US government's nutrition guidelines was overwhelmingly (more than 50 percent) comprised of people with ties to the food industry.[2] Lobbying groups influence research as well. A 2014 study published in the academic journal *Obesity* and authored by a leading "obesity" researcher found that drinking diet soda leads to more weight loss than drinking water.[3] The study was funded by a nonprofit group called the Global Energy Balance Network, which turns out to be a shell for Coca-Cola; the senior researcher was also a consultant for the soda giant.[4] This study is not unique. Between 2011 and 2015, ninety-six national health organizations accepted money from Coca-Cola, PepsiCo, or both.[5] Industry funding of nutrition research is commonplace.[6] A study concluding that eating oatmeal for breakfast keeps you fuller was funded by Quaker Oats.[7] Studies purporting the benefits of walnuts in diabetes prevention were funded by the California Walnut Commission.[8] Research hailing the use of grape juice in improving cognitive function is driven by the grape juice company Welch's.[9] An analysis of food-industry-funded research suggests that these studies were almost eight times more likely to report a favorable outcome for the industry than research that is not industry funded.[10] Another article concluded that over 92 percent of the industry-funded studies published in a year had results favorable to the funding source.[11]

The foods that are most demonized as "unhealthy" are those that low-income families (disproportionately BIPOC) tend to rely on, convenient energy-dense foods that efficiently feed a family on a tight budget. Sometimes it seems that the categorization of foods as "healthy" or "unhealthy" is based more on who eats them than on the nutrition content. Juice is a great example of this. In low-income areas, a carton of juice is affordable and easily accessible at the dollar store. This juice is largely seen as "unhealthy." A parent who pushes a stroller with a toddler sucking on a juice box may be given a nasty look or even called out as a bad parent. *Don't they care about the health of their child?* Media campaigns target low-income BIPOC, discouraging consumption of juice by warning of the increased risk for "obesity" and diabetes. It has even been suggested that low-income people be prohibited from using SNAP (Supplemental Nutrition Assistance Program, commonly known as food stamps) to buy juice and other sweetened beverages. But if you stroll over to a wealthy part of town, you'll see a juice bar on every other corner. These trendy beacons of health serve juices similar to what is looked down upon in low-income neighborhoods, but these juices—and the well-heeled people who drink them—are seen as virtuous and healthy with buzzwords like "cold-pressed" and "antioxidant." One glass of this "healthy" juice costs roughly four times as much as an entire half-gallon of "unhealthy" juice. Except for the price, presentation, and perhaps the presence of kale, there are few differences. The villainization of foods common in low-income communities, and their link to weight and health issues, contributes to further stigmatization of these groups, falsely portraying health as a matter of personal choice rather than systemic inequalities—for example, lack of access to adequate and inclusive medical care, and to affordable and well-stocked grocery stores, as well as the impact of chronic stress. In contrast, eating "clean," raw, or vegan becomes a status symbol for the overwhelmingly white wealthy elite. It is important to recognize where our belief systems about nutrition stem from and who is most harmed by them.

Cravings: Friend, Not Foe

All this outside nutrition advice has little to do with what our body needs. Diet culture robs us of our ability to feel competent in feeding ourselves. And this is exactly what diet culture wants—for us to be dependent on dieting and "experts" to tell us what, when, and how to eat. A narrative is set forth: If left to our own devices, we would eat ourselves sick and be utterly unable to care for ourselves. We must fight our cravings and try to outsmart our body. If we can just eliminate certain foods from our diet and "detox," our cravings will subside. If we do have a craving, we should distract ourselves with a brisk walk or warm bath and our cravings will pass. If we (gasp) give in to our temptations, we are undisciplined and lack self-control.

The irony is that it is the resistance, the fighting against our cravings, that makes our cravings feel overwhelming and out of control. When cookies are "bad," a craving for a cookie can send us into a panic. *How are we going to manage the craving? Will we be able to resist?* A test of wills is staged. *Me versus the cookie. Who will be the victor?* If we eat the cookie (which research shows we most likely will), our inner critic berates us. *You have no self-control. You shouldn't be allowed to have cookies in the house. You'll eat just a salad for dinner to repent.* Now food feels scarce. *I won't have cookies again. I'm going to have an unsatisfying dinner. I won't get to enjoy food again.* This can bring us into the screw-it mentality. *I've already blown it, one more cookie won't hurt. You have no self-control, you may as well eat the rest of the cookies or you'll be thinking about them all day.* Before we know it, we've eaten so many cookies that we feel sick and are more convinced than ever that we simply can't be trusted around cookies. But the cookies were never the problem. Trying to resist the cookies is what makes us feel out of control.

Research suggests that dieters have cravings that are more frequent, stronger, more difficult to resist, and slower to disappear when compared with non-dieters. In 70 percent of instances, dieters eventually "caved" and ate the foods that they were craving, although they reported less enjoyment of the food (guilt and conflict can really spoil the pleasure of eating).[12] In cultures where certain foods like chocolate are normalized and eaten regularly, such as in Spain, people report few cravings for chocolate. In the United States, where there is more prohibition and judgment around chocolate, it is one of the most commonly craved foods.[13] Remember, when we fight against our body, it's almost always a losing battle.

If you are feeling out of control around a certain food and/or binging on it, experiment with welcoming that food into your everyday life with abundance. For example, if you feel like you'll eat ice cream morning, noon, and night if left to your own devices, I encourage you to test that theory out. What happens when you have unrestricted access to ice cream? Next time you go to the grocery store, buy at least five pints of ice cream (if money and freezer space aren't concerns). Allow yourself to have as much ice cream as you want. This is not a test to see if you can keep the ice cream in your freezer without eating it! Or to see if you can have a small portion without losing control and eating more. I really mean it—eat as much as you want. If you go home the first night and eat so much ice cream that you feel sick, try to offer yourself compassion (and maybe some antacid). If you notice your inner critic telling you that you have failed, that you can't be trusted around ice cream, or that you were a fool to think that you could have this food in the house, simply observe and label this voice and try to ground yourself in the here and now, focusing perhaps on your breath for a moment or two, and ask yourself how you can move forward with compassion. Stay the course. Try to go out to the store as soon as is practical and replace however many pints you ate. Continue to allow yourself to have ice cream whenever you want. Continue to replenish your supply when it dwindles. Observe any harsh thoughts without letting them drive your actions. Over time, you may notice that the intensity of your feelings around the ice cream starts to diminish. It's no longer a test of wills or the forbidden fruit; it's just ice cream. Once its grasp on you has loosened, you can enjoy ice cream whenever you want it but also not think about it so much the rest of the time. You may even have times when you forget the ice cream is there!

Once you feel secure that you can eat what you want when you want it, you can start to focus on what you want and when you want it. We've already learned how hunger and fullness can guide us in when and how much to eat. Cravings, food preferences, and the way that our body reacts to different foods help us choose what to eat.

In the past, you may have gone through phases of "eating what I want" in rebellion of dieting. In those instances, rather than truly eating what we wanted, we instead only ate all the foods previously off-limits. It's more of an angry, screw-it mentality than a mindful attunement with our body. As we loosen the reins on restrictive eating, similar feelings may arise. We may go through a phase of wanting to eat only the foods that had previously been forbidden. This is only natural, because it can take time and experience to feel secure that we really can eat these foods as much as we want whenever we want them. As disconcerting as this may feel, try to allow yourself to eat what you want. Don't overthink the messages your body is sending you. Try not to judge your urges. The more that we fight against it and restrict ourselves, the more that we foster a sense of mistrust in ourselves and insecurity that food will be available to us when we want it. This drives us right back to diet mentality and the vicious cycle we are trying to escape.

Contrary to what diet culture teaches us, our cravings are important messages from our body that help us decide what we want to eat. Our body likes homeostasis, and when our nutrition (or gut microbiota, as we'll learn soon) is out of whack, our body may try to regain stability by encouraging us to eat certain foods through cravings. While the research results are mixed (and largely suggest that cravings are more heavily influenced by psychological deprivation than nutritional deficiencies), some studies suggest that when, for example, our body is low in iron, we may crave meat. When our blood sugar drops, we may crave sweets and simple carbohydrates to restore sugar balance. If our body is low on fatty acids, we may crave cheese, fried foods, eggs, or oily fish like salmon. Chocolate cravings may mean that we are low on certain vitamins and minerals contained in cacao or that our body needs more of the neurotransmitter serotonin (chocolate contains the amino acid tryptophan, a building block for serotonin), which is linked to antidepressant effects. When we have an urge for salty foods like chips or pickles, our electrolytes may be low or we may be dehydrated. Even cravings for nonfood items, a symptom of pica (an eating disorder where people crave and chew substances such as clay, paper, or soil), have been associated with a mineral deficiency. Research studies suggest that eating a diet low in variety is associated with more food cravings because our body is attempting to get nutrients needed from different food groups.

Cravings can even be driven by the bacteria in our bellies. For every one of our cells, it is estimated that we host ten microorganisms (in the gastrointestinal system it's more like 1:100), meaning we have 100 trillion teeny-tiny bacteria, viruses, fungi, and other creatures living in our body. The colony that lines our digestive system, the gut microbiota, plays an important role in digestive health and may influence what we eat. Each type of microorganism in the microbiota eats a different nutrient. For example, yeasts eat sugar, bacteroidetes feast on fat, *Prevotella* dine on carbs, and *Bifidobacteria* thrive on fiber. These colonies like to remain in balance; too much of one type of organism can throw our digestive health out of whack. When the organisms don't get enough food, the colony will dwindle. For example, on a sugar-free diet our yeast colonies may dip low, which leaves room for other colonies to grow unbridled. As a survival mechanism, the dwindling colony will send us signals through the gut-brain axis (the gastrointestinal system communicates with the brain through hormones released into the blood system and directly through the vagus nerve connecting the gut and brain), prompting us to eat the foods it needs. The microbiota may trigger cravings by changing our taste buds, increasing reward receptors, and producing neurotransmitters serotonin and dopamine (our natural antidepressants) to reward us for eating the foods the microbes need. If we don't eat what we are craving, the microbiota can also make us feel lousy by producing toxins as they die off.[14]

In a study looking at fruit flies, researchers found that when they manipulated the gut bacteria, the flies chose different foods based on their gut microbiota.[15] Similarly, studies of specially bred germ-free mice (with no microorganisms) found that these mice have altered taste receptors on their tongues that change if you give the mice microbiota, indicating that the microbes affect food choices.[16] In humans, gastric bypass surgery changes the gut microbiota, and people report corresponding changes in cravings after surgery. Pregnancy also alters the microbiome, and researchers think that these gut organisms may be responsible for the unusual cravings that people experience during pregnancy. Researchers have even found different microbial metabolites in the urine of people who love chocolate compared with people who are indifferent to it, despite both groups eating the same diet, indicating that the microbes may be triggering these yearnings for chocolate.[17]

While sometimes cravings are driven by what our gut needs, other times our cravings are triggered by what our brain needs. Cravings can be driven by monotony, a likely contributor to the increased cravings experienced by dieters. In a research study that fed people a boring diet of a nutritionally complete sweet liquid supplement, participants reported a significant increase in cravings.[18] Specifically, participants craved entrées and foods that had a different sensory quality than the liquid diet they were being subjected to in the study. They did not have increased cravings for sweets (the liquid they were given was sweet), which highlights how cravings are affected by regular access to foods. But most diets prohibit sugar and, unsurprisingly, dieters commonly report cravings for sweets.

Cravings can also be driven by certain emotional states. When we feel depressed, we often crave carbohydrates, a macronutrient that boosts our levels of serotonin (a neurotransmitter with antidepressant effects linked with mood stabilization and improved sleep). Chocolate, another commonly craved food when we are feeling down, contains alkaloids that also raise serotonin levels.[19] When we feel stressed, we may be more likely to crave salty foods, which have been shown to reduce the stress hormone cortisol.[20] Cravings are tied to the areas of our brain linked with pleasure and memory, suggesting that our desiring certain foods is related to our past experiences of these foods as pleasurable and wanting to have that nice experience again. Remember that when we eat foods that our body finds pleasurable, it shifts us into the rest-and-digest parasympathetic nervous system, decreasing stress and allowing us to relax. It's incredible that when we are feeling down or stressed, our body triggers us to eat specific foods to help us feel better. Not even my best friend knows me on that level! Many of us yearn for someone to sense our needs and care for us unconditionally; this is exactly what our body is trying to do.

Our Body's Response to Foods

Mindful eating doesn't end when we've swallowed our food. Our body continues the digestion process by breaking down our food into nutrients to feed our cells (and our microbiome). As you process the food you've eaten, you will likely notice that different foods have different effects in your body. For example, a big plate of broccoli may make you feel gassy. A big bowl of pasta may make you tired afterward. A candy bar may give you the quick boost of energy that you need to stay alert in an important meeting. Or the same candy bar may cause your blood sugar to crash, triggering a headache. A turkey and cheese sandwich at lunch may give you the energy you need to get through the afternoon, while a salad leaves you feeling worn out. Or vice versa.

What foods make you feel best vary by individual. The pizza that powers up your coworker could leave you running for the toilet (especially if you are lactose intolerant). The salad that satisfies your spouse at dinner may leave you feeling hungry. Your best friend swears that your sushi lunch makes her sleepy, while you feel full of energy. We each have different bodily needs. The key is to tune in to how certain foods make you feel with a sense of curiosity and compassion. Think of each eating experience as a learning opportunity to further explore what your body needs to feel its best.

If you find there are certain foods that your body doesn't tolerate well and you want to keep these foods in your eating repertoire, you may want to experiment with different ways of eating them and seeing how your body responds. For example, some people find that a food that makes them feel sick when eaten in large quantities is better tolerated when eaten in smaller portions. I want to note that I'm talking about food tolerances here, not food allergies. If you are allergic to a food and you don't eat it, then you don't need to reintroduce it. If you have a food allergy and want to experiment with reintroducing the food, that should only be done under the guidance of a medical professional. Food combinations impact digestion too. If a candy bar makes your blood sugar crash when eaten alone, eating the candy along with protein (peanut butter, anyone?) may slow the digestion of the sugars and avoid the crash. We are often quick to write off our favorite foods—*I always feel sick when I eat ice cream*—but we can explore ways to eat these foods that feels better. Whenever possible, think of nutrition in terms of adding foods in rather than taking foods away. Of course we may find that some foods just don't sit well with us, or we may have food allergies or intolerances and choose not to eat certain foods.

Unrestricted eating doesn't mean that we must eat all foods or eat foods that don't make us feel good. Quite the opposite, it's about choosing what foods we enjoy most and make us feel our best. But it's important that this be a choice we make, not a prohibition. How our body reacts to different foods is a piece of information we can use when deciding what to eat. Let's say that every time you eat a large meatball sub, you feel so sleepy afterward that it's hard to keep your eyes open. When deciding what to eat for lunch, after doing a mindful pause, checking in for hunger and fullness, and asking yourself what you want to eat, the meatball sub comes to mind. You are hungry, it sounds enjoyable, and you are in the mood for the flavors. But you know you have an important meeting this afternoon; you want to feel energized and alert. So perhaps you decide that you are not going to have the meatball sub now, but if you are still in the mood for it later, maybe you'll have it for dinner. Just because the sandwich makes you feel sleepy doesn't mean you can never eat it. It simply may be reserved for times when the sleepiness is a price you are willing to pay to eat the sub. Similarly, if you know that eating onions gives you gas, and you see the onion soup on the menu while you are out on a hot date, you may decide that, even though the soup sounds delicious, you don't want to worry about farting all evening, so you order the lobster bisque instead, which also sounds appealing. You may decide to eat onion soup the next night, when you'll be staying home alone.

Some foods may rarely seem worth it to us because the price is higher than the return. For example, if you feel sick every time you eat a hot dog, and it isn't a food you really love anyway, you may rarely choose to eat a hot dog. Hot dogs may become even less appealing because you associate them with the discomfort of feeling sick. Chocolate, on the other hand, may be worth eating, even though it sometimes triggers a migraine, if it's one of your favorite foods. But you may be more selective about what kinds of chocolate you eat and when you eat it, holding out for a truffle from your favorite chocolatier at a moment you are really craving it and can lie down and rest if a headache does ensue. It's all about moment-to-moment choices, not restrictions or prohibitions.

Mindful Eating and Chronic Health Conditions

If you have a chronic health condition such as diabetes, hypertension, or celiac disease, you may wonder if you can practice mindful eating. *How can I eat what I want if my doctor told me I can't eat sugar/salt/gluten?* Doctors often make sweeping recommendations to avoid entire food groups without understanding how the different foods in those groups impact your unique body. Which makes sense—doctors tend to be busy folks and don't know how each food affects each individual, so they err on the side of more restrictive recommendations to avoid all the foods that *may* impact your health condition. Unfortunately, medical professionals often don't recognize the risks and ineffectiveness of restrictive dieting, so what seems like a benign recommendation can send people down a rabbit hole of dieting, overeating, guilt, and shame. The shame that comes with breaking a medically recommended diet is particularly insidious because we are taught that it means we don't care about our health.

We must remember that our body is wise. Even if it's not functioning exactly the way we want it to, it is doing its best to keep us alive and will send us signals to help us care for ourselves. Let's take diabetes as an example. Diabetes is a condition where it is difficult for the body to regulate glucose. People with diabetes are often advised to eliminate all sugar and many carbohydrates from their diet, leaving them grasping at a restrictive diet with no white bread, white rice, dessert, or even fruit. As we already know, this kind of diet is nearly impossible to sustain long-term. And for people to manage their diabetes, it is not always necessary. To understand what our body needs, one of the most important things we can do is listen. Our body does a pretty good job at letting us know how it tolerates different foods. For example, if a person with diabetes has high blood sugar (hyperglycemia) after eating a certain food, they may feel symptoms including fatigue, headache, increased thirst, increased urination, and blurred vision. If a person with diabetes has low blood sugar after eating a certain food, they may feel symptoms like shakiness, sweatiness, dizziness, weakness, chills, and a fast heartbeat (among other symptoms). Blood sugar monitoring can help them tune in to their body, using a device such as a continuous glucose monitor or manually checking their blood sugar. They may find it helpful to use these devices in concert with mindfully checking in with their body, so they can start to sense what it feels like in their body when the monitor registers a high or low blood sugar.

Similarly, if a person who has celiac disease (an autoimmune disease where your body produces an immune response to gluten) eats a food with gluten in it, such as a piece of bread, their body will send out loud and clear signals that this is a food they can't tolerate. After eating gluten (sometimes amounts as small as crumbs), someone with celiac disease may experience symptoms including diarrhea, bloating, gas, abdominal pain, nausea and vomiting, constipation, and fatigue. Someone who has lactose intolerance is unable to digest the sugars in milk and may experience diarrhea, gas, and bloating after eating dairy products.

In many ways, mindful eating with a chronic health condition isn't much different from any other mindful eating. Your body provides valuable information that can guide your eating. If your body doesn't tolerate a certain food well, this becomes a piece of information you can use when choosing what to eat. Remember, this is always a choice, not a prohibition, even if your body doesn't tolerate a food well. If you have diabetes and you know that each time you eat cake your blood sugar goes high and you feel lousy afterward, you factor this into your decision. Is the cake worth feeling lousy afterward? Try to ask this without judgment; there likely will be times when it is worth it (e.g., a slice of cake from your favorite baker in a moment where you are really craving dessert and you have some time to rest and recuperate afterward, along with a plan discussed with your doctor to take any extra medication if needed) and times when it isn't worth it (e.g., a slice of cake that's not your favorite flavor in a moment when you don't particularly desire anything sweet and you have important activities afterward).

As discussed earlier, if there are foods that you have difficulty tolerating but want to keep in your diet, or you find yourself binging on them if you try to eliminate them from your diet, you can experiment with eating the foods in different amounts and in combination with different foods to see if that affects how your body takes these foods in. Working with a weight-inclusive, Health at Every Size–informed dietitian can be invaluable in helping you parse how different foods affect your body and ways to use your body's own guidance to care for your chronic health conditions.

It's also okay not to eat certain foods that don't make your body feel good and/or don't work with your health condition. Some people misinterpret *allowing* ourselves to eat all foods as meaning that we *have to* eat all foods. This of course is not true. For example, if someone with celiac disease experiences intense pain each time they eat gluten and has sustained a gluten-free diet for several years without it triggering episodes of binging on gluten, there is no need for them to suddenly start eating gluten just because they are practicing mindful eating. If what you are doing is working for you, feel free to continue that path. But if you have a food intolerance and find yourself binging on that very same food you are trying to restrict, it may worth examining if restricting that food is the best path for you.

In many chronic health conditions, what we eat only accounts for some of the management strategies, even though our culture would have us believe otherwise. As we learned in chapter 2, factors such as genetics, access to health care, discrimination, marginalization, and stress play big roles. Don't let diet and exercise be the only focus in managing your chronic health condition. For example, in diabetes, stress can make it more difficult for your body to regulate glucose. This means that people who are under high stress—whether an isolated event or a chronic condition—may experience more high and low blood sugars even when eating similarly to someone with less stress. Trying to follow a restrictive diet, being hard on yourself when you can't sustain that diet, coping with internalized weight bias, and living in a world where you face chronic marginalization and discrimination can all impact stress and consequently blood sugars. While we can't meditate our way out of systemic oppression, a mindfulness practice can help us develop better ways to cope with chronic stress and mitigate its impact on our health. It can also give us more resiliency to advocate for change in the societal structures that are affecting our health in the first place.

When you come up with a treatment plan with your doctor, it is important to accept your current style of eating and base your treatment on that. Yes, in theory, if you never eat another carb, eat no sweets, including fruits, and basically sustain yourself on kale and quinoa for the rest of your life, you may be able to avoid going on medications for your diabetes. But this isn't realistic for most of us. We know that restrictive dieting tends to lead to out-of-control eating. Your body doesn't care if you are dieting to lose weight or because your doctor told you to; it just knows it is being deprived and will rebel. When there are medications available that can help you manage diabetes effectively while eating in sustainable ways, what is the point of torturing yourself on a plan that isn't sustainable only to beat yourself up when the plan inevitably fails? If you have diabetes and you eat carbs, work with your doctor to manage your diabetes while eating carbs. If you love oranges, try to incorporate them into your treatment plan. Your doctor's job is to develop a care plan that will work for you as you are, not you in some alternate version of reality!

How to Make a Mindful Choice

When choosing what we want to eat, we can be guided by our hunger, fullness, taste enjoyment, food preferences, cravings, body's reactions to foods, and practicality. Before eating, try these steps to play with making mindful choices:

1. Take a mindful pause for hunger and fullness. How hungry are you? How full are you? Do you want to eat right now? If you are hungry, what foods will satisfy your level of hunger? For example, if you are just starting to experience the mildest symptoms of hunger (a 1 on the Hunger Scale) and you know that you have dinner plans in an hour, you may decide that a muffin or some cheese and crackers could be a satisfying snack. If you are very hungry (a 3 on the Hunger Scale), you may choose a more filling meal. Or if you are very hungry but know you will have dinner soon, you may choose to eat something small to reduce your hunger but leave some hunger remaining for your dinner. If you are not hungry (0 on the Hunger Scale) but sitting down for dinner with friends, you may choose to order something small to nibble on so you can participate in the meal, or order something that you will enjoy eating for leftovers in case you don't want to eat it all now. Remember, it's all about what you want to choose—you absolutely can eat a large meal if you are mildly hungry or a small snack if you are very hungry; there is no right or wrong here!

2. Now expand your awareness to notice if there are any foods that you are drawn to in this moment. What do you want to eat? Is there anything you are clearly in the mood for? Any cravings for a specific food? What sounds enjoyable right now?

   If nothing specific comes to mind, consider tastes, flavors, textures, or temperatures. If you can't think of a specific food, you may notice you are in the mood for something crunchy or salty or spicy or with mayonnaise. You may want something hot and comforting on a cold day or something cold and refreshing on a hot day (or vice versa). You may want the flavors of Indian food or Southern or Thai.

3. How do you want to feel after eating? Are you looking for a meal that will leave you energized and refreshed? Or are you planning to lie down and relax after eating? If you already have a food in mind, consider how this food has made you feel in the past. If it's a food that your body tends to not tolerate well, are you willing to feel that way after eating? Again, there is no right or wrong here. If you are lactose intolerant and in the mood for ice cream, you may be willing to spend the evening sitting on the toilet if you don't have any other plans and are really excited for a sundae. But if you are about to go into an important meeting with your boss to ask for a big promotion, you may not be willing to risk having to make a mad dash to the bathroom.

4. What foods are available to you right now? If you are having difficulty deciding what to eat, you may want to consider some readily available choices and see if they seem appealing. What foods do you already have in your house? If you have some leftover baked ziti in the fridge, along with the shrimp stir-fry you made for dinner last night, and the fixings for a sandwich, do you want any of those options? If a sandwich shop, salad store, and pizzeria are all convenient options, check in with yourself to see if any of those choices seem appetizing.

No matter how much we work to increase food availability, there are always going to be some limitations. For example, if you are getting ready to eat and notice you are craving the duck à l'orange from Le Petit Canard in Paris, getting on a plane to France for dinner may not be entirely practical. But is there a way to satisfy your craving within the confines of the food that is available to you now? Is there a similar dish at a local restaurant? Would Peking duck from your favorite Chinese restaurant fit the bill? Or perhaps putting some orange marmalade on the roast chicken in your fridge? Are you wanting the memories of that special time in Paris? If so, perhaps look at photos from your trip. Or find the recipe of the dish online and plan a special night to cook and enjoy the meal. Similar situations may arise if you are craving a food that doesn't fit your budget. Try to get creative and think about ways you can best approximate meeting your needs, even if it's not an exact fit.

5. If you notice judgment or diet thoughts driving your food decisions, observe these thoughts, label them ("diet thoughts," "judgment," "inner critic," "the patriarchy," etc."), and try to shift your awareness back to the information you are gathering from your own body. Judgments around food can be stubborn and deeply ingrained. I swear that WW plants a point-tracking chip deep within our brain that can take decades to deactivate. Our hands may reflexively turn a package over to consult the nutrition label when deciding if we want to eat something. Remnants of diet culture are sure to remain, even when we are dedicated to working from an anti-diet approach. Don't give yourself a hard time. Simply notice, label, and ground yourself back in the present moment with the knowledge that these thoughts are no longer serving you and you have the wisdom within to care for yourself.

TAKE-ACTION ACTIVITIES

See how your body reacts

Notice how different foods affect your body. If you want, experiment this week with keeping a journal of what you eat and how you feel afterward. Do certain foods give you more energy? Do other foods upset your stomach? Make you feel lethargic? This can be especially useful if you struggle with health issues that may be exacerbated or eased by certain foods. If writing down what you eat feels too reminiscent of food logs from your dieting days and you think it could bring up more dieting mentality, I recommend skipping this activity.

Have a mindful meal out

It doesn't have to be anywhere fancy—whatever seems appealing and fits in your budget. When you arrive at the restaurant, take a mindful pause for hunger and fullness. Then expand your awareness to see what you are in the mood to eat. Does anything immediately call your attention? Any specific flavors, textures, or temperatures that seem appealing? How do you want to feel after eating? Next look at the menu. Peruse it leisurely, reading every item, even dishes that you would typically pass over. What seems appealing to you? What best aligns with what you are in the mood to eat, what you think you would enjoy, and how you want to feel after the meal? Do you notice any diet culture thoughts trying to interfere with your decision of what to eat? If so, observe, label, and try to gently refocus back on the wisdom of your body.

When your food arrives, take a moment to do another mindful pause for hunger and fullness. Has your hunger or fullness changed at all? Examine your food with your eyes, and observe as much as you can about its appearance. Smell your food and notice any aromas. What on your plate do you want to try first? Put your first bite of food in your mouth and notice the taste. Give yourself a rating on the Taste Enjoyment Scale. After you swallow the food, do you notice your body responding to this food in any way? Lead yourself through the process of eating your meal mind-fully, choosing each bite of food, using your senses to observe as much as you can about the food, giving each bite a rating on the Taste Enjoyment Scale, noticing how your body responds to the food, and checking in with your hunger and fullness and noticing how your ratings on the Hunger Scale and Fullness Scale change as you eat. Notice the point where you feel satisfied and no longer want to continue eating. Do any feelings arise?

Practice mindful cooking

Think about what you would like to make. What seems fun to prepare? What might be enjoyable to cook? If you don't like to cook or don't have access to a kitchen, consider preparing a cold dish like a sandwich or salad. Stroll through a local market and get inspired by fresh ingredients, or recreate a childhood favorite. If you notice diet culture thoughts come up while deciding what to make, simply notice, label, and shift your focus back to connecting with your body and the task at hand.

Try to bring your mindfulness skills to every aspect of the cooking experience, looking at the appearance of the ingredients, smelling the ingredients, and noticing the texture. How do the ingredients transform as you start cooking? Are there sounds from cutting the food and pre-paring it for cooking? What about sounds as you are cooking? Do aromas emerge as you are cooking? When your meal is finished, how do you want to present it? As the saying goes, we eat with our eyes first. How can you plate the meal so it looks most appetizing?

As you prepare to eat the food you've cooked, take a moment to think about how all the ingredients on the plate came to be here and how they have combined to create this dish. Lead yourself through the process of eating your food mindfully. Can you taste each ingredient in the dish?

Eat mindfully from many choices

Family-style meals and buffets are fantastic opportunities to experiment with making mindful choices. Next time you are presented with a bunch of food choices, take a moment to look at each item offered. At a buffet, this may mean taking a walk around it to see all the options before putting food onto your plate. What seems most appealing? Do you want to sample a food you don't usually eat? What are you in the mood to eat? How do you want to feel afterward? Check in with hunger and fullness and think about what may be satisfying. Take the foods that you want on your plate and eat them mindfully, checking in with taste enjoyment, hunger, and fullness.

Notice how your body reacts to the food. What foods do you enjoy and what don't you care for? Are there any foods that you want more of? Any on your plate that you don't want to finish? When you are finished eating, think about if there is anything else you want to eat. Do you want a second serving of any of the items? Anything you didn't try that you want to taste now? If you want, go back up to the buffet or food table and take more food. Lead yourself through the process of eating it mindfully, and repeat until you feel satisfied and choose to stop eating.

Explore abundance

If you struggle with feeling out of control with certain foods, experiment with welcoming those foods in abundance. As instructed in this chapter, if you worry that you will eat a certain food morning, noon, and night if you let yourself, test that theory out. Allow yourself to eat that food whenever you want it and in whatever quantities you desire, perhaps keeping a stock of it in your home, and see what happens. For example, if you feel out of control with ice cream, load up your freezer with five pints. Worry about eating too much chocolate? Buy several king-sized bars. Feel like you would eat chips nonstop? Stock your pantry with a bunch of family-size bags and see what happens.

If you eat "too much" of the food at any point, stay the course. If you overeat, offer yourself comfort and compassion. If you feel sick after overeating, consider if there is anything you could do to make yourself feel better. Perhaps some mint or ginger tea to soothe your tummy or changing into some comfy clothes and lying down with a heating pad? Try not to let any incidents of overeating or feeling out of control deter you from continuing this exercise. As soon as you say, *See, I can't be trusted around this food, I can't keep it in my house!* and go back to restricting it, scarcity mindset takes the driver's seat and you are more likely to feel out of control. Observe any thoughts of restriction and judgment that may come up during this exercise, including thoughts like *it's okay to eat this food, as long as I don't eat too much* or believing that this exercise is a test to see if you can have the food in your house without eating it. As much as possible, try to keep your stock of the food in good supply. When you've eaten some of the food, try to replace what you've eaten as soon as is practical.

Maintain your meditation

Continue to meditate for three, five, ten, or fifteen minutes daily. You can either set a timer and practice independently—walking yourself through the process of focusing on your breath, noticing when your mind wanders off, and gently bringing your awareness back to your breath—or listen to the guided meditations available at www.drconason.com/diet -free-revolution/. You are also welcome to experiment with using the many guided mindfulness meditations available online or on different apps. Remember: if you are struggling to set up a consistent daily practice, you can always revisit chapter 3 for more guidance.

9

STEP 9: Learn to Manage Emotional Eating with Compassion
How to Give Yourself What You Really Need

I t was a Wednesday evening in late February and the weather had turned bitterly cold. A thin layer of frost covered my office window, giving the street below the appearance of one of those perfect little holiday villages that people display on their windowsills at Christmastime. Despite the cold outside, my office felt warm. The heat purred in a rare moment of cooperation when it wasn't sweltering or freezing. Tracy, Linda, Michael, and Mia gathered in my office, each assuming the seat that had become "theirs" during the group. Mia and Linda sat together on the couch (now Mia relaxed into the seat, allowing herself to take up the space she needed), Michael was in the club chair on the periphery of the room, and Tracy sat in a folding chair between them. On a few occasions, Mia noted that it seemed unfair that Tracy was always stuck with the least comfortable seat in the room. She offered her spot on the couch, but Tracy always declined, saying she preferred the folding chair. I wondered if Tracy would say if she wanted to switch. It was hard for Tracy to advocate for herself, whether she wanted a more comfortable chair, onions left off her meal at a restaurant, or more support from her husband.

Asserting herself with her husband was particularly difficult. Her marriage was challenging, to put it mildly. "I know that I'm stuffing my feelings down with food," she said. In one of our earlier individual sessions, Tracy had disclosed that she thought her husband was having an affair. Despite her husband's betrayal, Tracy blamed herself for the breach in their marriage. "I've let myself go. This isn't what Jay signed up for when he married me." I wondered if anyone really knows what they are signing up for when they get married; isn't that kind of the point? Jay's appearance had also changed in the fifteen years they had been married—after all, aging and body changes are some of the few certainties in life—but Tracy didn't fault him for this the way she held her own body accountable.

When Jay and Tracy first married, they strived for an egalitarian marriage. Both were progressive thinkers who rejected traditional gender roles. They committed to an equal division of household labor. Each worked a demanding job, Tracy in publishing and Jay in finance, and in the early days of their marriage, it seemed easy to divide the housework equally. But as the years went on, the tides shifted. At first it was Jay, the better cook of the two, neglecting dinner duties when he worked late. Tracy readily picked up the slack, having dinner ready when Jay got home. Then Jay got a coveted promotion, which made late hours the norm, and Tracy also took over the laundry. After all, she reasoned, she got home earlier, and Jay was working so hard—and earning the bigger paycheck now—it made sense for her to do more housework. She started to feel indebted to him as he was now paying most of the bills and financially supporting their lifestyle. It wasn't long before Tracy assumed the bathroom cleaning and eventually litterbox responsibilities for Jay's cat, Seymour, a wretched animal from Jay's bachelor days that snipped at Tracy whenever she came near. Things spiraled fast when Madison was born. A simple calculation showed that they would spend more on childcare than Tracy's yearly salary. Jay's prospects at his brokerage were hopeful and far more lucrative than Tracy's publishing career. Begrudgingly, Tracy quit her job to care for Madison. She told herself it would just be for a few years; once Madison started school she would refocus on career. But when Liam was born four years later, her hopes of returning to work became even more far-fetched. Fifteen years into their marriage, Tracy was loath to realize they had fallen into the same traditional gender roles they had hoped to avoid; Jay was the sole income earner, and Tracy took care of everything else.

Tracy hardly had time for herself. Days were spent shuttling the kids to school, sports practices, music lessons, dentist appointments, and play-dates. She became an afterthought in her own life. While the kids always had a satisfying packed lunch and snacks, Tracy would stave off hunger by grabbing the fastest, most convenient food possible, giving little thought to what she truly wanted. She hadn't bought new clothes in years. *What's the point in spending money on new clothes when my body looks like this?* Tracy felt acutely uncomfortable in her skin. Each morning when she dropped her kids off at school, she dreaded seeing the other mothers. All svelte and polished, with their hair blown out and designer workout clothes, they huddled outside the classrooms talking about things like anti-aging treatments and flab-busting fitness routines. Tracy couldn't help but compare herself and feel she didn't measure up. Her curly hair didn't hold a blowout, and she wouldn't dare wear the revealing spandex outfits the other moms looked so at ease in—even if they came in her size. Surely Jay would be happier if he had married one of them. *It's my fault that he has strayed.*

Tracy and Jay were like two ships passing in the night, sharing a home but little else. Jay was obsessed with work. He left for his office early in the morning and returned late at night. When he was home, notifications from emails, texts, and phone calls were incessant. He retreated for hours on end into his home office, emerging only for a bite to eat or, in the evenings, to refill his scotch glass. Recently Tracy noticed the muffled sounds coming from behind the closed office door sounded more intimate than professional. There was laughter and conversations that seemed to last for hours. She found unusual charges on his credit card bill, expensive dinners from nights he said he was working late and charges from a jewelry store when he never gave her jewelry. Sex went from infrequent to not at all. Tracy didn't dare confront him with her suspicions. She was terrified of what he would say. Not that he would confirm the affair—she already felt certain it was happening—but that he would say *why* he was cheating. That he would admit her body repulsed him.

With Jay sequestered in his office and the kids asleep, evenings were unbearably lonely. Food helped ease the pain. Bowls of cereal, ice cream, and cookies punctuated the long hours. Exhausted from taking care of everyone else all day, Tracy took care of herself this way. She could do whatever she wanted. Eat what she wanted. Watch what she wanted on television. Mindlessly scroll through social media. But this way of taking care of herself came with a darker side—her harsh inner voice chastised her for eating this way, for looking this way, for being this way. As she cleaned up the dishes before bed, hoping no one would notice the missing food, a wave of sadness would wash over her. *What has my life become?* She would cry herself to sleep, tears soaking the silk pillowcase they had received as a wedding gift more than a decade earlier.

"Does the food help you?" I asked Tracy. She looked at me, trying to gauge what I thought her response should be. "There's no right answer," I assured her. Tracy answered back, "While I'm eating, it feels good. It's enjoyable. It takes me away from the sadness and comforts me. But then I feel sick. And I get so mad at myself. I end up feeling worse than when I started."

The other group members were all nodding their heads. "That resonates," I observed. "Yeah," Mia jumped in, "that's totally my experience too. When I'm eating, it's like a high. It feels awesome. But, man, the crash is hard. It provides some relief in the moment, but after I've eaten I feel even worse. All I can think about is how gross I feel."

Evenings were tough for Mia too. It had been a few years since she first moved to New York, but she was so busy with work that she hadn't made many friends. How do you make new friends as an adult anyway? New York, and all the glamour that surrounded her, made her feel like an outsider. Mia shared a one-bedroom apartment with three roommates who had subdivided the space into tiny parcels to give each their own room. Her bedroom, just large enough for a twin bed and small dresser, was her refuge. She felt safe hidden away from the outside world and dreaded having to leave her room to use the bathroom or go to the kitchen, journeys that took her across the living room where her roommate Bri would be sprawled out on the couch with her boyfriend in varying stages of undress. *They must think I'm such a loser, always home alone, never out with friends, never on a date.* Although Mia had profiles set up on all the dating apps, she was constantly deleting and reinstalling them on her phone. She yearned for a partner but became overwhelmed with self-criticism each time a swipe didn't pan out or, even worse, at the prospect of actually having to meet someone in person.

Food provided comfort during the dark nighttime hours. Each night, she would pick up food on her way home and bring it into her room, trying to hide the large take-out bag from her roommates. She didn't want anyone to notice what or how much she was eating. Once she was safely in her room, she would change into her comfy pajamas, set up her computer to stream episodes of whatever show she was engrossed in, and sit on her bed with the food, eating straight from the take-out cartons with plastic utensils. She ate slowly, drawing the experience out over multiple courses as she watched her shows. When she had eaten all her food or couldn't fit any more in her stomach, a wave of sadness would wash over her. Her enjoyment for the night was done, and now the despair rolled in. She curled up on her bed with a bellyache and stared wistfully out her window at the building across from her. Each little box was aglow with life, and Mia couldn't help but imagine the warm scenes behind the curtains—perhaps a family eating dinner together, a parent helping a child with nightly home-work, a couple watching the evening news on the couch. It was all so banal but felt a world away as Mia lay in her dark bedroom alone. *I'll never have that. Who would ever love me, especially when my body looks this way?* It didn't take long before Mia turned back to the familiar refrain of hating her body.

"Maybe that is one of the ways that eating helps you cope with difficult emotions," I said. "After you eat, you focus on how sick you feel, or beat yourself up for having eaten, or obsess about much you hate your body. As uncomfortable as these feelings may be, they are familiar. They feel more manageable than deep loneliness or whatever else you are feeling.

Historically, we believed we have control over feelings around food and our body. If eating is the problem, then we can just eat less. If our body is the problem, we can just lose weight. It's an easier solution than the messiness of our emotions. Pretty amazing all the ways that food can help us cope."

Food can help us through some difficult times. Throughout my years as a therapist working with people struggling with eating issues, I've heard many stories of clients who turned to food in the immediate aftermath of trauma. Children and teens who had their first binge episodes after they had been violated, suffered grave loss, had their view of the world turned upside down, felt alone and unsafe. People who soothed overwhelming emotions with food, sought moments of pleasure in times of bleakness, and found a way to survive. The resiliency of humans never ceases to amaze me. To use food to cope is a sign of strength and perseverance. I know in my own life food has gotten me through some tough times. And I'm incredibly grateful for that.

Unfortunately, in diet culture emotional eating is maligned, seen as a sign of weakness and failure rather than resilience. It is something to gain control over, overcome, and conquer. We internalize these beliefs, shaming ourselves for using food as a source of comfort. This turns emotional eating into a double-edged sword where it is simultaneously rewarding and punishing. For many people, emotional eating is distressing—not because of the eating itself but because of the harsh self-reproach that follows. It is imperative that we change this narrative around emotional eating. Remember, as we learned in chapter 4, punishment does not lead to change. Beating yourself up for emotional eating will not make you stop emotional eating. It will only make you feel more stuck, helpless, and miserable. True change comes from acceptance, nurturance, compassion, and love. Eating is not a moral characteristic; we are not "good" when we eat in response to physiological hunger and "bad" when we eat in response to emotions. What would it be like to see emotional eating not as a shortcoming but as a miraculous sign of resilience? To have gratitude toward food for shepherding you through times of difficulty? To embrace experiences of emotional eating without judgment?

What Is Emotional Eating?

What do you picture when you think of emotional eating? Most of us envision eating to soothe sad, anxious, stressed, or angry feelings. This is what we often see portrayed in the media: a woman crying into a pint of Ben & Jerry's after a breakup, or a woman anxiously nibbling her way through a bowl of chips while waiting for her date to call. We can thank romantic comedies for these highly gendered, heteronormative associations of food as a replacement for love. But emotional eating is far more expansive. For the purposes of this book, I define emotional eating as any non-hunger-based eating (that is not medically prescribed, as in the case of someone in recovery from an eating disorder or managing a health condition). This may include eating to comfort ourselves in times of sadness or anxiety, eating for the pure act of pleasure (dessert, anyone?), eating for celebration (birthday cake!), eating as a cultural norm (not wanting to offend your neighbor when they offer a home-baked scone even though you aren't hungry), and much more.

Emotional eating is a completely normal and healthy part of being human. We all eat emotionally at times. If we didn't, we would eat birthday cake only when we were hungry, few of us would take a second (or third) helping of Grandma's special Thanksgiving mashed potatoes, and family trips to the ice cream parlor after eating a full dinner wouldn't exist. Healing our relationship with food does not mean eliminating emotional eating. Rather, it means making choices about when we want to eat for nourishment, for comfort, for soothing, for connection, or for the pure experience of pleasure. These are all completely valid choices, but they are just that—*choices*—rather than reactive, compulsive, conflicted, disconnected, out-of-control behaviors that we then beat ourselves up for afterward. My hope for you is that emotional eating becomes a choice that you embrace without judgment and serve up alongside heaps of self-compassion.

As Mia shared in her example, eating until we feel physically sick and then berating ourselves for overeating can serve a purpose as well. As uncomfortable as this part of the cycle is, it is familiar and may feel more manageable than the emotions that triggered eating in the first place.

When we eat so much that we feel physically sick, feeling sick becomes the problem—our focus centers on our physical discomfort, not our underlying emotions. When we berate ourselves, our problem becomes the way we eat and the way our body looks—which can feel more manageable because we believe it has a solution (just control our eating, go on a new diet, try a juice cleanse, take the latest pills), whereas coping with other feelings can feel amorphous and overwhelming. How many of us have comforted ourselves from the despair following a binge with thoughts of a new diet plan? Unfortunately, as we are learning, this way of thinking only keeps us stuck in the cycle we are trying to escape.

Think back to a time where you ate emotionally. It may be a difficult period in your life when you relied heavily on food, it may be a specific incident that stands out in your mind, or it may just be a recent time you ate emotionally, perhaps earlier today or within the past few days. Whatever comes to mind, try to envision this experience as fully as possible. Picture where you were, what you looked like, what you ate. Are you aware of what emotions triggered you to eat? How did you feel while you were eating? How did you feel after eating? Did you treat yourself with kindness and compassion or harshness and criticism? Now bring your awareness to your breath for a few breath cycles, taking a moment to center yourself in the present moment. Then envision yourself again after that time of eating emotionally. This time imagine bathing yourself in self-compassion. Visualize treating yourself as you would treat a beloved child, friend, or pet who is going through a difficult time. How might you comfort them? How can you help them feel loved and cared for? What would that look like? Can you apply this to yourself? What would be some words of kindness that you can offer yourself? What could you do to nurture yourself? Can you thank food for helping you through that time of difficulty?

Next time you find yourself eating emotionally, try to recognize any tendencies to fall into habitual patterns of self-criticism. When you notice self-criticism arise after emotional eating, pause, observe, and label these thoughts ("criticism," "judgment," "Ruby," "diet culture internalizations," etc.). Focus on your breath for a moment, and try to move forward with compassion. Express gratitude for how food helped you. Did it soothe you, numb you, relax you, or shift you into the parasympathetic rest-and-digest nervous system? Did it give you a moment of pleasure? Accompany you through a tough moment? Food is a valid coping mechanism that is always available to you. Can you extend the gratitude toward your body? Perhaps thanking your body for being able to digest the for food, for breathing, and for keeping you alive? It may feel nice to place a warm loving hand of comfort on your belly or another place on your body that needs soothing. Try to treat yourself like a precious loved one.

Throughout your journey, please remember that emotional eating is always available to you. No one ever has the power to take that away. When you need it, you will find it there, just as it has always been. But you may find that as you practice the methods suggested in this book, your relationship with emotional eating will change. Rather than something to be fought against and met with shame, it becomes a tool you can utilize compassionately, without judgment. We will also learn how to use other tools to nurture our emotions. As amazing as food is, it is not a one-size-fits-all solution. Our emotional needs are diverse, and food simply can't do it all. You deserve to have your emotional needs cared for in the most complete ways possible.

Three Steps to Working with Emotional Eating

Over my years of working with clients, I have developed a simple three-step process to work with emotional eating. But just because something is simple does not mean it is easy. There is a reason that we've been using food to cope with our feelings; our emotions can be messy and hard to deal with. Here's the good news: you can do hard things. Just look at what you've already accomplished on this journey! You are moving away from the dieting paradigm that you've relied on for so much of your life, venturing out on new ground, learning to trust your body when you've been indoctrinated to believe you need to fight against it, and taking a leap of faith. Here are the three steps:

1. Identify your hunger. Do a mindful pause for hunger and give yourself a rating on the Hunger Scale. Eat if hungry. If not, move on to step 2.

2. Identify your emotions. What are you feeling?

3. Meet your emotional needs.

Let's dig into each step in more detail. The first step is to understand if your urge to eat is being driven by physiological or emotional reasons. Remember, both are equally valid reasons to eat. Food is the only thing that can satisfy physiological hunger, but there are many ways that we can satisfy our emotional needs. To assess if you are physiologically or emotionally hungry, do a mindful pause for hunger (see chapter 5) to give yourself a rating on the Hunger Scale. If you are hungry, eat. If you have the urge to eat and are not physiologically hungry (0 on the Hunger Scale), this is a clue that your desire to eat is being driven by emotions; move on to step 2. There may be times that you notice your urge to eat is driven by both emotions and physiological hunger. In these moments, it is important to eat to meet your hunger needs. And if there are emotional needs to be met, you can work to satisfy these as well after you are fed.

If you aren't physiologically hungry and have the urge to eat, step 2 is to identify any emotions that you are experiencing. This can be challenging, especially if we've spent most of our life turning away from our feelings. It may be helpful to think of the basic emotions that psychologists have identified: happiness, sadness, fear, and anger (some also include disgust and surprise). Like the primary color wheel, these emotions can combine to create additional emotions. For example, anger plus disgust equals contempt. Happiness plus surprise equals delight. If you are having difficulty identifying your emotional experience, use these basic emotions to see if any of them match what you are feeling.

Emotions are experienced in both mind and body. When we experience an emotion, our brain triggers a reaction in our body to prepare us for anticipated events. For example, fear triggers muscle tension and rapid heart rate so we can run as fast as possible to escape danger. The way we speak about emotions highlights these bodily connections; for example, we can experience "heartbreak," "cold feet," "butterflies in our stomach," and "a gut feeling." A 2014 research study revealed that bodily experiences of emotions are universal across cultures.[1] Anxiety commonly manifests as tightness in our chest, gastrointestinal distress ("a nervous stomach"), pounding of our heart or rapid heartbeat, sweating, and trembling or shaking. Anger can show up as tension in our neck, shoulders, arms, and hands (especially clenched fists), increased heart rate, and feelings of hotness in our face ("hot-headed"). Sadness is associated with a heavy feeling in the chest ("a heavy heart"), a sinking feeling in the stomach, and decreased sensations in the legs and arms. Happiness is a full-body experience, triggering a symphony of sensations from our head to our toes including feeling warm, relaxing of our muscles, and, of course, smiling. We can use our physical sensations as clues to identify our emotions.

It's nearly impossible to identify our emotions if we don't give ourselves the space to check in with ourselves. Try a mindful pause for emotions to increase awareness of your feelings. (These instructions can also be found in the Take-Action Activities at the end of this chapter.) Bring yourself into a meditative position with your feet flat on the floor and your spine upright, or whatever posture your body is calling for at this time. Bring your full awareness to your breath for a few breath cycles, noticing your breath as it enters and exits your body. Then gently expand your awareness to your entire mind and body. Are there any emotions that rise to the surface? Any physical manifestations of emotions that you are aware of? Any thoughts or mental manifestations of emotions? Where in your body do you feel your feelings? Try to label your emotions. It can be useful to recall the basic emotions (anger, disgust, fear, happiness, sadness, and surprise) and see if any of these emotions can name what you are feeling in this moment. Feel free to use emotions outside of that list as well if any come to mind. If you can't identify what you are feeling, that's fine too. Be patient and gentle with yourself; this can be challenging! Just differentiating physiological hunger from emotionally driven hunger is a huge first step.

After you have identified and labeled your emotions, it's time to move on to step 3: meeting your emotional needs. Sometimes there is a clear path to addressing emotional needs; for example, if we are feeling lonely, perhaps connecting with a friend could tend to these feelings. When we are anxious or angry, diaphragmatic breathing (also called "belly breathing," a process where we breathe so our belly expands on the inhale and contracts on the exhale) can help calm our body and nudge our nervous system out of fight-or-flight response into rest-and-digest. Some people find that writing their anxieties down on paper (a "worry list") can help calm their mind. Releasing energy through physical activity, like in a kickboxing class, punching a pillow, or progressively relaxing any clenched muscles, may help disperse anger.

But often there is not a clear solution to our feelings. In these cases, what we really need is to allow ourselves to experience our feelings. In a culture that encourages us to avoid uncomfortable feelings at any cost, sitting with our emotions can feel downright bizarre. We have mistakenly been taught that it is possible to get through life pain-free. That we can enjoy the excitement, happiness, and joy without the worry, anger, and sadness. Just take in the good things and leave the bad behind. Strong or negative emotions—especially if we dare to express them—reveal personal shortcomings. If you struggle with difficult feelings, you haven't mastered the life hack to unlock unlimited happiness. Of course, none of this is true. That life hack doesn't exist, and uncomfortable emotions, along with pleasant ones, are a natural and unavoidable part of life. To be human is to suffer *and* to have joy. Mindfulness encourages us to welcome in the full range of emotional experiences without pushing away, holding on to, or judging them. This process of fully embracing life—warts and all—is what Jon Kabat-Zinn calls "full catastrophe living."

Emotions are like waves in the sea. They build up, crest, break on the shore, and retreat. This is the natural life cycle of emotions. When we try to keep our emotions at bay, however, the natural ebb and flow can be interrupted. What if, rather than allowing our emotional waves to naturally break ashore, we build a dam to hold the water away from the land? The water accumulates behind the dam, becoming more and more forceful, until it eventually breaks through the barrier and a tsunami comes barreling toward us. The torrent of water is terrifying. We want to run and take shelter to protect ourselves. When we consistently turn away from our emotions, we create a barricade to keep them at a distance. This can be exhausting to maintain, and when it eventually gives way, the cascade feels overwhelming. While it may feel like the *emotions* are overwhelming, often it is the *barricade* that is most formidable. Without the barricade, our emotions would gently roll in and out.

In Buddhism there is the teaching of the two darts. As we go through life, we inevitably get hit with "darts." These darts are events that cause us pain. Getting hit with the first dart is unavoidable; we will all go through painful experiences in life. When many of us get hit by the first dart, however, we immediately get struck by a second dart. This second dart is our reaction to the pain—the narratives we create about the pain, the mental maneuvers we ineffectively perform to avoid the pain, the fear and anxiety about the pain, and our feelings of judgment, guilt, and criticism. This dart is avoidable; when we accept the first dart, we don't get hit by the second one. The Buddha taught that the first dart causes pain, the second dart causes suffering.

Often it is the second dart that is most distressing. The story of our pain—rather than the pain itself—torments us. We try to avoid our feelings because we fear what we *believe* them to be rather than what they are. The narratives we create around our emotional experiences overwhelm us. We worry that if we allow our feelings in, we will never be able to escape them. But the reality may be very different. It's like a child afraid of the dark. In their room alone at night, the abyss under their bed becomes a fertile environment for a monster. The child lies in bed terrified, imagining the worst-case scenarios in their mind. Eventually they call out for their parent or caregiver, who (in an ideal situation) comes to comfort the child. The adult turns on the lights and allows the child to see what is truly there.

What was imagined to be the monster's furry claw is just some crumpled laundry on the floor or a misplaced teddy bear. In the light, what the child feared turns out to be mundane.

What would you see if you shined a light on your feelings? Our emotions are important messengers of information, wisdom that we can glean from our internal well of knowledge. Emotions tell us when something needs tending to, and if we listen to our feelings, they can lead us toward deeper ways of understanding and caring for ourselves. Turning away from our emotions may lead to neglect of parts of ourselves and feelings of deprivation. Fighting against our emotions may also lead to them seeming more overwhelming, like in the barricade analogy we discussed earlier. When we welcome our emotions in, they say what needs to be said, express themselves, and leave.

Imagine that a visitor comes to your home. Perhaps it is your landlord looking to collect rent or your neighbor coming to gossip. You're not in the mood to see anyone, so you ignore the knocking at the door and pretend you aren't home. But your visitor will not be easily deterred. They knock louder. They start calling your name. *I see your car out front! Are you home?* You hear them walking over to a window and jump into a closet to hide. Through the narrow slats of the closet door, you see their face pressed against the windowpane. They are knocking on the window now, the glass vibrating with the force. *I know you are in there. I see your coffee on the table and your jacket is still on the hook. Are you trying to avoid me?* They shuffle around to your back door and beat heavily on the outer door. *Let me in!* They are shouting now and shaking the flimsy screen door. It doesn't take long before they realize the back door is unlocked and angrily come barging into your home.

While you may have delayed seeing this person, hiding from them was stressful and now the situation has escalated. How might this have been different if you had warmly greeted them at the front door and invited them in for a cup of tea? Even though you don't want this person to be here, they are indeed at your door, and ignoring them only seems to make the situation worse. Greeting our emotions is a form of acceptance; whether or not we want these feelings to be here, the reality is that they are here. We can't make the feelings go away, but we can decide how we want to react to them. Do we fight against them (build a barricade or hide in the closet), or do we welcome them in (let the ebb and flow be uninterrupted)? As an aside, this analogy only works in reference to our emotions. With actual people who are trying to barge into your home, boundaries (and locking your door) work wonders.

Our mindfulness practice is an entry point for increasing awareness and acceptance of our feelings. Becoming present and checking in with our internal experiences give us the space to recognize our feelings. This may start with noticing feelings that arise during our formal meditation practice. There have been many times that I sat down to meditate feeling tuned out, only to be gifted during the practice with the awareness that my mind was being carried away by thoughts of worry, sadness, excitement, or another emotion. I closed the practice with a newfound insight that I had feelings that needed tending to. The mindful pause for emotions (which we learned earlier in this chapter) can help us focus our awareness specifically on our emotional experiences occurring in our mind and body. If you notice emotions arise, experiment with allowing yourself the space to fully feel your feelings. If you notice a narrative arise around these feelings (*these feelings are bad, I shouldn't feel this, get it together, don't cry*, etc.), simply observe this narrative, take a moment to center yourself by focusing on your breath for a few breath cycles, and refocus your awareness on the emotional experience. Treat yourself with compassion. Remember, difficult emotional experiences are a natural part of the human experience—you are not alone. How can you best care for yourself at this time? If it's useful, think of a small child or animal that is suffering. How would you treat this being that needs your comfort, soothing, and love? Can you offer yourself what you would give to another?

If your emotional experiences feel overwhelming or difficult to cope with, it is important to seek therapy with a licensed mental health professional. While pain in life is unavoidable, suffering is not. We don't always need to take the most challenging path, and there is no virtue in suffering needlessly. You don't have to go through this journey alone. Psychologists, social workers, marriage and family therapists, mental health counselors, psychiatrists, and other mental health professionals are trained to help you navigate difficult emotional experiences. While emotions ebb and flow, psychiatric disorders are more persistent. For example, sadness may come and go over the course of a few hours or days, but depression typically persists for two weeks or more. If you are struggling with a mental health condition or your emotions feel intense, volatile, and difficult to manage, I strongly encourage you to seek support. You can find a list of therapists who identify as weight-inclusive providers at www.drconason.com /diet-free-revolution/. You can also search therapy listing sites such as www.PsychologyToday.com to look for local providers. Many of these sites have search features that can filter by location, specialty, and what insurances they accept in-network. If you are looking for a therapist in-network with your health insurance plan, your insurance company can provide a list of local therapists. Community mental health clinics often provide low-fee or sliding-scale services. Training clinics (often part of universities or postgraduate programs) offer lower fees along with the opportunity to work with a student-therapist who is under the supervision of a more experienced licensed therapist—two minds for the price of one! I'm of the mindset that most people can benefit from having someone to talk with, and we don't have to hit rock bottom to get support. If you are wondering if therapy can help you, I encourage you to give it a try.

Takeaways

We all eat for emotional reasons at times, whether it is celebrating a birthday with a slice of cake, munching on chips when we feel stressed, or prolonging the pleasure of a delicious meal with a second serving even though we aren't still hungry. Emotional eating is a normal part of the human experience. If you find yourself turning to food for emotional reasons, try to offer yourself compassion. Observe and label any self-critical thoughts that may arise, reminding yourself that they are just thoughts, not the truth, and try to move forward with kindness.

While food is one way to cope with our emotional needs, it is not always the best way (even food can't do it all!) and can sometimes lead us to push away, rather than turn toward, our feelings. Using the techniques you learned in this chapter, you can identify your emotions and choose the best ways to tend to them; sometimes that may be actively doing something (like calling a friend or moving your body), sometimes it may be leaning in to your feelings and fully experiencing them, and other times it may mean choosing to eat. The intention is that this becomes a mindful, conscious, and aware choice that you make with your own best interests at heart.

TAKE-ACTION ACTIVITIES

Gratitude exercise for emotional eating

How has emotional eating helped you in your life? Has food been a way to cope in times of difficulty? Has it comforted you when you needed comforting? Brought you pleasure when things felt bleak? Numbed you when you were overwhelmed? Helped you persevere and survive? Journal (or just think) about the ways that emotional eating has served you in your life. Can you foster a sense of gratitude for emotional eating? Can you appreciate the ways that it helped you get through those difficult experiences? What are some ways that you feel grateful toward food?

Gratitude meditation for emotional eating

Bring yourself into a meditative position, sitting in a comfortable upright seat with your feet flat on the ground and your spine upright, or whatever position your body is calling for at this time. Start out by focusing on your breath, bringing your full awareness to your breathing for a few breath cycles, noticing the inhale and exhale, staying completely present with this current moment. If at any point your mind wanders off, simply observe this and gently refocus your awareness back on the task at hand. When you are ready, bring to mind a time that you ate emotionally. It may be a difficult period in your life when you relied heavily on food, it may be a specific incident that stands out in your mind, or it may just be a recent time you ate emotionally, perhaps earlier today or within the past few days. Whatever comes to mind, try to envision this experience as fully as possible.

Picture where you were, what you looked like, what you ate. Are you aware of which emotions triggered you to eat? How did you feel while you were eating? How did you feel after eating? Did you treat yourself with kindness and compassion or harshness and criticism? Try to remember this experience in as much detail as possible. When you have done so, return your awareness to your breath for a few more breath cycles, anchoring yourself back in the current moment in the safety and comfort of your breath. Then envision yourself again in that emotional eating experience. But this time imagine bathing yourself in self-compassion. Feel yourself being immersed in love and kindness. What does that look like? What does that feel like? What are some words of kindness that you can offer yourself? How can you nurture yourself? Can you thank food for helping you through that time of difficulty?

Honor the resilience within you for finding this tool to cope. Try to foster a sense of gratitude to food for all it does for you and to yourself for finding powerful ways to comfort and care for yourself. When you are ready, return your focus to your breath, grounding yourself back in the present moment for as long as you need. When you are ready, bring the practice to a close.

Mindful pause for emotions

Bring yourself into a meditative position with your feet flat on the floor and your spine upright, or whatever posture your body is calling for at this time. Bring your full awareness to your breath for a few breath cycles, noticing your breath as it enters and exits your body. Then gently expand your awareness to your entire mind and body.

Are there any emotions that rise to the surface? Any physical manifestations of emotions that you are aware of? Any thoughts or mental manifestations of emotions? Where in your body do you feel your feelings? Try to label your emotions. It can be useful to recall the six basic emotions (anger, disgust, fear, happiness, sadness, and surprise) and see if any of these emotions can be used to name what you are feeling in this moment. Feel free to use emotions outside of that list as well if any come to mind. If you can't identify what you are feeling, that's fine too. No matter what your experience is, be patient and gentle with yourself. It can be hard to identify our feelings, especially when we've spent so much of our life trying to turn away from them. Just starting to recognize that an emotion is present, even if we can't exactly name it, is an important step.

Practice these three steps when you have the urge to eat

Step 1: Identify Hunger. Give yourself a rating on the Hunger Scale. If you are hungry, eat food. If you are not physiologically hungry, move on to Step 2.

Step 2: Identify your emotions. Do a mindful pause for emotions, and label any feelings that you notice.

Step 3: Meet your emotional needs. How can you best care for yourself in this moment? There is no one right answer here; it is about making a choice that feels compassionate, nurturing, and attuned to your feelings. For example, you may decide to connect with a friend if feeling lonely, rest if feeling tired, or cry if feeling sad. Choose to lean in to emotions and experience them fully if that feels right to you in the moment. Or you may choose to eat to soothe your emotions if that feels most nurturing. Whatever you choose to do, try to do it without judgment. If you notice judgment arise, simply notice this, label it (e.g., "judgment," "inner critic," "Tim"), and return your awareness back to your breath for a few cycles before reengaging with this process.

Journal about your experiences practicing these three steps—what was happening in your mind and in your body?

Maintain your meditation

Continue to meditate for three, five, ten, or fifteen minutes daily. You can either set a timer and practice independently—walking yourself through the process of focusing on your breath, noticing when your mind wanders off, and gently bringing your awareness back to your breath—or listen to the guided meditations available at www.drconason.com/diet -free-revolution/. You are also welcome to experiment with using the many guided mindfulness meditations available online or on different apps. Remember: if you are struggling to set up a consistent daily practice, you can always revisit chapter 3 for more guidance.

10

STEP 10: Live a Life Full of Self-Care, Pleasure, and Value

It was a few minutes before the start of our final group session, and behind my closed office door I could hear Tracy, Michael, Mia, and Linda chatting in the waiting room. Michael was getting a new ferret to keep Buddy company. He was starting to date a bit and worried that Buddy was lonely now that he wasn't spending as much time at home. I could hear them all cooing as, I could only assume, Michael showed them pictures of the creature on his phone. I was struck by how close the group had become, four people with worlds of differences between them. If they had met at a cocktail party, it's hard to imagine the conversation would've lasted more than a moment. But in this setting, where they spoke about what lies below the surface, they were bound by the universalities of feeling not good enough and the shared goal of escaping that suffering.

I opened my door and invited everyone in to start the session. As they filtered into my office, the jovial mood from the waiting room shifted. "I don't feel ready to end," Mia said with trepidation after taking her seat. "It seems like we are just getting started." The other group members nodded in agreement. "It *is* just the start," I confirmed. "Think back to how long you've been struggling with your relationship with food and your body. In context, our time together is just an instant. The purpose of this program was never to get you across the finish line. It was to set you on a new path. To give you tools for your journey forward."

It is unrealistic to heal lifelong issues with food in just a couple months. By the final group session, however, no one was dieting anymore. While some did experience the urge to diet every now and again—especially when they were targeted for advertisements for programs claiming to help you lose weight without dieting (spoiler alert: it's a diet)—these urges were now recognized as internalizations of diet culture, not as truths to be followed. Many of the group members continued to grapple with body image, especially as some experienced changes in their bodies. It was clear to all, however, that the key to improving body image and coping with these changes in their body was changing their mindset, not changing their body. For some, that process included mourning the loss of the body that they wished they had—or perhaps even had embodied at an earlier time in their life. Their mindfulness practices helped them sit with and explore their complicated feelings about their body (chapter 3). To cope with judgments and shame that arose around their body, the group members used the skills they had learned for labeling self-criticism (e.g., "internalized weight bias," "judgment," or "patriarchy"), centering their awareness on the present moment (i.e., focus on breath), and finding a way to move forward with compassion (chapter 4). While they didn't always like their body, they were learning how to more peacefully coexist with it. They were all committed to following the path toward trusting their body, even if that path was treacherous at times.

We spoke for a bit about the progress each had made in the group. Linda was coming to peace with her body, slowly accepting that it would never be the same as it was when she was twenty years old. She grieved the loss of her younger body but also explored ways to best care for the body she was in. She discovered tai chi and practiced with a local group weekly, enjoying both the movement and the community. She made regular trips to her favorite bakery and savored her buttered toast in the morning, no longer viewing carbs as the enemy. She could keep bread in her house now and didn't feel compelled to eat it all at once; she took some when she wanted it and didn't think about it otherwise. She enrolled in the pain-management program at a top-notch hospital, where, as previously mentioned, she began physical therapy and acupuncture to seek relief from her chronic pain now, in her current body. Professionally Linda considered the next phase of her career. She shifted her perspective from seeing the younger generation of associates at her office as the enemy and took on a mentorship role. She discovered a sense of purpose and meaning in passing down all that she had learned in the business. She looked for ways that she could slow down and enjoy the life that she had worked so hard to build for herself.

In the spirit of the fat acceptance movement, Tracy came to embrace the term *fat* as a descriptor for her body. Reclaiming the word dissipated her fears that her husband would name it for her. The more that she acknowledged the reality of her body—yes, she was fat—and worked to question the narrative that it was bad and shameful, the more compassionate and accepting she felt toward herself (even if she didn't always like the way that her body looked). As the pervasive shame lifted, she felt empowered to address the issues in her marriage, and she and Jay were getting ready to start couples therapy. For the first time in decades, Tracy wasn't binging regularly. She wasn't fighting against it, but it just kind of lost its appeal. She ate what she wanted when she wanted, and without the restriction to rebel against, the binges were anticlimactic. When she did binge (which happened occasionally), she leaned into the episodes, allowing herself to binge, and was kind to herself afterward. This made the binge eating feel less upsetting, the episodes were less intense, and she moved on from them more easily. Tracy started to find sources of pleasure in other areas of her life: painting and dance were two pursuits that she now prioritized making time for, after years of them being pushed out because of her caring for others.

Michael was spending less time at the gym and starting to explore the world of dating, even taking a body-positive course about online dating for extra support. He bought some new clothes that fit his current body and cleared out his closet, donating older clothes that were too small. While it was hard to let go of the fantasy that he would get back into these smaller clothes (items he had bought the year after his surgery when his body was smaller than it had ever been, even as a child), he found freedom in the flexibility and expansiveness of his current life. He became playful with fashion, exploring what helped him feel both confident and comfortable. Michael still enjoyed a good workout, but the gym became a "want to" instead of a "have to" and wasn't the centerpiece in his life. He was still apprehensive about dating—especially sex—but he yearned for a partner and was able to tolerate and work with his discomfort as it arose, using some of the skills we learned in chapter 9.

Mia decided to leave her job working for the fancy designer, in search of a better quality of life. She was on her third round of interviews at a small up-and-coming plus-size fashion company known for its supportive work environment. She no longer relied on coffee to dampen her appetite in the mornings and found that eating a satisfying breakfast did a much better job of energizing her and powering her through to lunch. She reallocated her latte budget to grocery shopping and came up with satisfying lunches that she could bring from home, which allowed her to eat in a timelier fashion when hunger struck; even if she was busy, she could grab her lunch from the office fridge, whereas previously she would have delayed eating because she didn't have time to go out to get something. But despite all the progress Mia had made, something still loomed on her mind.

"This may sound silly," Mia said, "but without dieting, I feel lost. It was such a huge part of my life. It's how I knew if I was good or bad. I had something I was working toward, a clear way to improve my life. Without it, I'm floating untethered. Although it's not perfect, I feel so much better about my body and eating. But sometimes without dieting, I just think, *Who am I?*"

"It can be hard," I empathized, "to reconfigure our life without the structure of dieting. It's been a set of rules to live by, and there is comfort in that, even though it ultimately makes us feel trapped. Moving away from dieting can leave a void. But that space is full of potential—it's an opportunity to examine what is most important in our life. What values do we ascribe to? What gives our life meaning? What brings us joy, pleasure, and satisfaction?"

Viktor Frankl, an Austrian psychiatrist and Holocaust survivor, believed that humans are primarily driven by a need to make meaning of our life.[1] His work was informed by his experiences in the Nazi concentration camps, where he witnessed people finding meaning in the most dire of circumstances. In contrast, Sigmund Freud, the founder of psychoanalysis, believed that humans are driven by the "pleasure principle," a basic instinct to seek pleasure and avoid pain.[2] In my opinion, both pleasure and meaning are essential human needs. In 1943 psychologist Abraham Maslow theorized that we have a hierarchy of needs.[3] He grouped our needs into a pyramid with different levels and argued that we can't focus on our higher-level needs at the tip of the pyramid until we have met our basic needs that lie at the base of the pyramid. If our basic needs are not met, we become preoccupied with meeting those needs, and psychological illness or distress may result. In Maslow's model, basic needs are physiological ones like food, water, and sleep. Above that are needs for safety (which includes financial security and health), love and belonging, esteem, and self-actualization. The model is useful in illustrating how diet culture narrows our life. When we are consumed with what to eat, what not to eat, and if food will be available to us, we stay focused on meeting our most basic physiological needs. When we free ourselves from diet culture, trust that we can satisfy our hunger needs, and feel secure around food, we can expand our focus to other needs. These may include other basic needs like sleep, safety, and health, as well as higher-level needs like relationships, community, seeking pleasure, and living in accordance with our values.

Unfortunately, not everyone has equal access to fulfilling their basic needs, because of systemic inequalities like poverty and discrimination. For example, we can do everything in our power to break free from dieting, but if we aren't able to afford the food that satisfies our hunger needs, we will understandably remain preoccupied with this basic need for food. Food insecurity inherently means that there is not unrestricted access to food or a feeling of security that food will always be available, which may be some of the reasons that we see high levels of eating disorders and disordered eating in food-insecure populations who rely on a food pantry for meals.[4] If you can't afford a home, you will be focused on meeting your need for shelter. Illness and lack of access to health care will understandably keep us absorbed with our needs for bodily safety. Having unmet basic needs doesn't necessarily preclude you from meeting higher-level needs. In fact, Maslow emphasized that the hierarchy of needs is not a rigid order. But if basic needs are unmet, there is a lot more that you are dealing with, and understandably, resources will be directed toward what is needed most for survival. For those of us who do have the privilege of meeting our basic needs, we can consider working to increase equality for those who don't have these privileges. There is no easy solution here, but social justice work can be a starting point in addressing some of the changes we want to make in the world. One of the most powerful things about freeing ourselves from diet culture is the clarity we gain to stop focusing all our energy on shrinking our bodies and reallocate our attention and resources to the causes that are most important to us and our communities. We'll be talking more about living in accordance with our values later in this chapter, but first we have a few more basic needs to cover.

Self-Care 101

We live in a culture that teaches us to put ourselves last. Especially for those of us raised as girls, we are socialized to be quiet, caring, and self-sacrificing to prepare us for our expected roles of wife and mother. We are taught to be attuned to others' emotional experiences and tend to those above our own. Although we have made a lot of progress in the past several decades creating space for women in the work world, this has led to a demand that we "do it all" in both the work *and* domestic spheres—what sociologist Arlie Hochschild called "the second shift" in her 1989 book by the same name.[5] To be successful in the work world, women are expected to devote 110 percent to work and not take any concessions for personal needs. While a stay-at-home mom may deny her own needs to prioritize those of her children and spouse, a working woman may deny her own needs in service of the needs of the company she works for (and the larger system of capitalism that it is embedded in), and a working mom will be expected to prioritize the needs of her company, her children, *and* her spouse before her own. We work (whether paid or unpaid labor) to uphold the very same capitalist patriarchal systems that oppress us.

When we are given permission to care for ourselves, it's often only in the context of enhancing our ability to perform the roles demanded of us. Think about one of the most common self-care mantras: *put on your own oxygen mask first before assisting others*. While this may be useful advice in a plane crash, when it comes to self-care, the refrain only emphasizes how prioritizing our own needs is most valuable in the service of others. Self-care is also often couched within the patriarchal framework of making ourselves more appealing objects for others; for example, framing time dedicated to maintaining a slim figure as "taking care of yourself" or an extreme plastic surgery makeover as a means of "self-care."

Audre Lorde, acclaimed writer, activist, and self-described "Black, lesbian, mother, warrior, poet," said, "Caring for myself is not self-indulgence. It is self-preservation, and that is an act of political warfare."[6] In a culture that teaches us that our value is in self-sacrifice, self-care is an act of resistance and rebellion, not selfishness. It is also, as Lorde suggested, an act of self-preservation, especially for marginalized groups. Research suggests that self-care is fundamental to our health and well-being.[7] Caring for ourselves fosters resiliency and fills up our proverbial gas tank. In contrast, when we are exhausted and depleted, we are running on empty. We have few emotional resources to meet life's challenges. Any curveball that comes our way feels overwhelming.

Imagine the following two scenarios: In the first one, you wake up feeling exhausted. You stayed up too late finishing the season of your favorite show and then tossed and turned for most of the night. When your alarm starts going off, you hit snooze until you are running late. Frenzied, you forgo a shower and throw on the first clothes you can find, even though they are a bit too small and pinch your belly. You feel self-conscious but don't have time to change. Your tummy is starting to grumble, but there's no time to stop and eat. On your way to your meeting, you get a coffee. This is a necessary pit stop. You order your favorite double espresso latte and walk back to your car. You drive a few blocks before reaching a red light and finally taking a sip of your coffee. Yuck—the barista got your order wrong and gave you some horrid mint mocha concoction! Imagine how you might feel. How would you cope with the order mix-up? Do you feel angry? Frustrated? Helpless? Do you want to throw the coffee on the ground and stomp on the cup? Does it bring you to tears? Do you create a narrative that nothing ever goes right for you, that you must have the worst luck in the world? How might this event impact the rest of your day?

Now imagine a similar scenario, except this time you got a good night's sleep and wake up feeling well rested. You eat a satisfying breakfast, take a shower, put on clothes that you feel your best in, and do your meditation practice. On your way to your meeting, you stop for coffee. You order your favorite double espresso latte and walk back to your car. You drive a few blocks before reaching a red light and finally taking a sip of your coffee. Yuck—the barista got your order wrong and gave you some horrid mint mocha concoction! Imagine how you may feel now. Do you feel better equipped to cope? While disappointed, are you able to take the mix-up in stride without it derailing you? Does it still bring on the torrent of emotions that it did in the first scenario, or does it feel manageable when you have more resources to navigate the situation?

Most of us can cope with the coffee fiasco better in the second scenario because we have filled our tank with self-care (well rested, nourished, showered, comfortable, and meditated); when something doesn't go our way, like the coffee mix-up, we have more emotional resources to cope. When our tank is already on empty (tired, hungry, unshowered, uncomfortable, and rushing), we are just one latte incident from being pushed over the edge.

Many (perhaps most) of us are perpetually running on empty. Our needs don't get met and we feel deprived, uncared for, unseen, undervalued, and alone. We are last on our list. It is often not until the end of the day, after we have given it all to our jobs, kids, partners, pets, and everything else, that we finally turn our attention to ourselves. At this point we hardly have anything left to give ourselves. We are more likely to turn to things like food, alcohol, marijuana or other drugs, online shopping, television, social media, online gaming, or browsing the internet to tune out from rather than tune in to ourselves. There is nothing inherently problematic about most of these things (although any can be problematic with overuse; if you think you may have a problem, I encourage you to consult with a mental health professional), but consistently tuning out can lead us to further neglect our underlying needs and creates an endless cycle of depleted resources, feelings of deprivation, more tuning out, and so on.

For our purposes, we can think of self-care in a few different categories, which we'll call basic self-care, joyful movement, pleasure, leisure activities and social connections, and living in accordance with your values. These needs don't exist in a rigid hierarchy, and we don't necessarily need to fulfill them in any particular order; but our basic self-care needs almost always take priority, and if these needs are not satisfied, it can be harder to focus on the others.

Basic Self-Care

Basic self-care is tending to our most fundamental physiological needs. It includes things like sleep, hygiene, eating, drinking, physical comfort, shelter, and safety. Hopefully at this point we are all in agreement on the importance of consistently meeting our hunger needs. We have worked hard to feel as secure as possible that food will be available when we need it. Similarly, we need to drink hydrating liquids when we feel thirsty. It's commonly said that our body needs two liters (or eight glasses) of water each day. But this isn't completely accurate. According to the Centers for Disease Control and Prevention (CDC), the amount of water we need varies from person to person and is influenced by several factors including age, sex, pregnancy, and breastfeeding, as well as how much water we expel through sweating, urinating, and bowel movements (interesting fact: stool is mostly water).[8] We don't need to rely solely on water to meet our hydration needs and typically consume about 20 percent of our daily fluid intake from foods.[9] Fruits and vegetables, oatmeal, and soup are just a few examples of foods with high water content. Most beverages like iced tea, juice, and sports drinks contain a lot of water too.

Drinking when we are thirsty tends to be far less conflictual than eating when hungry. This is because we haven't been taught to mistrust our thirst signals the way we've been taught to mistrust hunger. When we are thirsty, we pour ourselves a drink with minimal thought. We trust our gut, with little interference from diet culture. When diet culture does infiltrate the world of beverages, people struggle more. For example, there is a lot of "obesity prevention" messaging around consumption of soda, juice, and other "sugar-sweetened beverages." Not surprisingly, when people do have conflicts around beverage consumption, it is these items they struggle with. Similarly, some diet programs encourage people to drink eight glasses of water per day (or more) to supposedly aid in weight loss. In this framework, it is not uncommon for people to criticize themselves and feel guilt and shame for not meeting these water-intake goals. Without fatphobia and diet culture, would our relationship with food look more like our relationship with water? When we felt a hunger pang, would we get up and get a snack as instinctively as we get a glass of water?

Sleep is another basic need. The CDC recommends that adults get a minimum of seven hours of sleep per night, and the National Sleep Foundation estimates we need between seven and nine hours a night.[10] The specific amount of sleep required varies from person to person, so it is important to listen to your body to see how much sleep you need to feel well rested and function optimally. According to the CDC, more than one-third of adults in the United States don't get enough sleep (which they define as less than seven hours per night).[11] About 40 percent of adults in the US struggle with daytime sleepiness severe enough to interfere with daily activities.[12] This lack of sleep can impact us physically and emotionally. It is associated with psychological issues including depression, relationship problems, poor performance at work, and impairments in memory, attention, and decision-making.[13] It takes a toll on our physical health and is associated with lowered immune system, high blood pressure, heart disease, stroke, and diabetes.[14]

Many of us don't even realize that we are sleep deprived. We believe that we must be one of those rare people who can function well with very little sleep. But when we tune in to our body, we find that we are sleepy. If you find yourself relying on caffeine to get you through the day, getting sleepy during long meetings, or consistently falling asleep when meditating, these may be signs that you aren't getting enough sleep. If you notice that you are tired, sleep is the best match for this need. Many of us try to fight daytime sleep, either with caffeine or by eating something. While this may give a short-lived burst of energy, it's not going to truly recharge you. Getting a good night's sleep or taking a nap will.

Tips on improving sleep hygiene abound, and you have probably heard some of the common ones. Limit screen time before bedtime. Create a relaxing nighttime ritual, perhaps a warm bath and mug of hot milk or chamomile tea. Use lavender aromatherapy. Set a cutoff time with work (including checking email) well before bedtime. Go to sleep and wake up at the same time every day. Keep the bedroom for sleep and sex only. Don't keep a clock by your bedside. Listen to a boring, soothing podcast (there are ones specifically designed for this purpose) or nature sounds such as ocean waves. Meditate (perhaps you have even noticed improvements in sleep since starting this program!). If you are having a hard time getting to sleep, feel free to try these tips. Maintaining good sleep hygiene is never a bad idea. But for many of us, they won't "cure" our sleep deprivation. And that is because our problem isn't that we *can't* fall asleep, but that we don't *want* to.

When we spend our days neglecting ourselves, evenings can become precious "me time." After all our work is done, we've walked the dog, cleaned the dishes, put the kids to bed, and done everything else that needed doing, we turn our attention to ourselves. It's not uncommon to stay up late into the night watching TV, eating, scrolling our phones, and pursuing other ways of mindless relaxing. The thought of going to bed is off-putting; it means our scarce time for ourselves is over and we are that much closer to waking up and doing it all again tomorrow. Hopefully as we start to care for ourselves throughout the day—carving out time for pleasure and things that bring meaning and purpose to our life—this time in the evening may feel less essential.

It's not always possible to sleep more. If you simply can't get eight hours of sleep at night, scheduling a daily nap can help. While it's not a replacement for a good night's sleep, napping can help reduce sleep debt, some evidence suggests. Studies have shown that napping can improve cognitive functioning after sleep deprivation, although it may not impact negative mood.[15] If you are having difficulty with sleep, please consult your health care provider.

Another form of basic self-care is caring for our health and seeking medical care when we need it. Sadly, in the US health care is a privilege, only available to those with financial means, employment benefits, or who qualify for the limited government programs currently available. Even if they can access care, many people will be subjected to subpar, biased care because of weight stigma, racism, sexism, transphobia, and other systems of oppression. The medical system prevents many people from meeting basic health care needs, and we see the consequences in health disparities among marginalized groups.

If you can access competent health care, this is an important facet of self-care. It includes going to the doctor for preventive screenings, seeking treatment when you don't feel well, caring for your dental health with regular cleanings and examinations, and caring for your mental health by seeing a therapist or psychiatrist when needed. It also includes regularly taking prescribed medications and having conversations with your doctor if you are not consistently taking these medications for any reason. It may also involve additional forms of healing such as acupuncture, physical therapy, and massage therapy.

While this is not a comprehensive list, my hope is that it is a launching point for you to consider your basic self-care needs. Meeting our basic self-care needs is essential for our survival. If these needs are unmet, functioning in other areas may be sacrificed. For example, we can't think as clearly when we are hungry or exhausted. As our basic self-care needs are met, we shift our focus to other needs like joyful movement, pleasure, social connections, and living in accordance with our values. Our attention isn't necessarily drawn to these needs in the same way as our basic needs. For example, it's hard to ignore thirst, illness, or physical danger, but it's easier to disconnect from needs for movement, pleasure, and values. While we can survive without meeting these higher-level needs, it is very difficult to thrive without them.

Joyful Movement

Diet culture has ruined exercise. We subject ourselves to various forms of torturous activities in the noble pursuit of weight loss. In my dieting days, I remember forcing myself to go to the gym even though I hated every minute of it. The gym was a place to punish my body for misbehaving. I chose the most vigorous forms of exercise I could endure, with little regard to what I enjoyed. After all, I was there to lose weight, not have fun. I sweated through workouts to the uninspiring soundtrack of self-criticism that played on a loop in my head. *Go faster, you loser. Don't stop now, you are disgusting.* Not surprisingly, I tried to avoid the gym whenever I could, and it would never be long after starting a new regime before I called it quits. The gym was all-or-none and linked with dieting; if I wasn't following my diet, why go to the gym? If I couldn't go to the gym regularly enough to see "results" (read: weight loss), why bother at all? If I wasn't going to do an intense calorie-burning workout, what was the point? And if I wasn't going to the gym, I may as well "eat what I want" (read: everything prohibited on my diet, whether I really wanted it or not). When I didn't maintain my gym routine (or diet), I blamed myself, believing that I was unmotivated and lazy. The gym was just another cog in the diet–overeating–self-hatred cycle.

It took many years before I could connect with movement as a form of joy instead of punishment. It came after a couple sedentary years when I was in graduate school. My busy schedule didn't allow me to go to the gym regularly, and if I couldn't get there five days per week as a former personal trainer had advised, I wouldn't see the results I wanted, so I stopped going altogether. I was driving to school and sitting in classes most of the day, then sitting and studying most of the weekend. My body started to speak to me when I experienced sciatica pain shooting down my leg. A doctor recommended stretching and gentle activity. The idea of gentle activity was novel, as was the idea of movement as a way to soothe my body rather than punish it. I found my way to Nia class, a type of movement that combines martial arts, dance, and yoga. In my first class the instructor had us close our eyes and move our body in ways called by the music. I felt silly but also connected with my body as a partner, not an adversary. I had always avoided dance; somewhere along the way I decided I was "bad" at it and felt self-conscious when I tried to dance. But in Nia it didn't matter if I was good or bad at dance—everyone's body looked different, and each person had a unique way of expressing the movements, which helped the comparisons and self-consciousness dissipate. For perhaps the first time in my life, I was enjoying moving my body. My pain improved, and I found myself laughing in the classes and moving my body freely and playfully, in ways that I rarely allowed myself to do. This felt tenuous—I worried about getting tossed back into the body hatred that had always accompanied movement in the past. Cautiously, I started to explore other forms of movement that seemed enjoyable, like other dance classes and slow-moving yoga. I found myself doing these activities because I wanted to, not because I had to, similar to how I may want to spend my free time going to see a movie, knitting, or doing something else enjoyable for myself. They nourished not only my body but also my mind and spirit.

When our experiences with exercise have been couched within diet culture, it can be hard to envision movement being a source of pleasure. But the human body was built to move, and you may find that when you connect with movement as a source of pleasure rather than punishment, it can feel good. In this section we are going to explore some ways to bring movement into your life with joy and pleasure. Everyone is in a different place with movement, and there is no one right way of doing things. You may already have a regular enjoyable movement routine that works well in your life. You may struggle to incorporate movement in a way that doesn't feel punishing or like a chore. You may have mobility limitations or chronic pains that limit your movement. You may not want to move. Wherever you are, that is where to start.

Self-care is not a moral obligation. If adding movement into your life simply isn't something that you can do or want to do right now, that's fine too! It doesn't make you one iota less of a valuable human being because you aren't active. Because so many of us have a conflicted history with movement, it's not uncommon for harsh self-critical thoughts to arise here. If you notice this, observe and label these thoughts (remember, they are just thoughts, not a gospel we need to live by), and try to move forward with self-compassion. Return to chapter 4 for a review on this technique if needed. If you find yourself rebelling or resisting against the material in this section, or if it is triggering diet mentality to arise, I recommend moving forward to the next section in this chapter, "Leisure Activities and Social Connections," and returning to this section when the time feels right. And try to do so with compassion.

For those of you interested in exploring enjoyable movement at this time, take a moment to imagine what it would feel like to move your body for the sole purpose of feeling good. Do you have a sense of what that would be like? Can you picture yourself doing it? What do you see? If you are having difficulty imagining it, it may be useful to think back to experiences of joyful movement in the past. Perhaps this was a time in your life when movement wasn't connected with weight loss, before you learned that your body is bad, when you felt at home in your body. A time when your body was a vehicle rather than an obstacle. Some of us may need to think way back to our earliest childhood memories. It may be the joy you felt as a child running through the yard with friends playing a vigorous game of tag, swinging from the monkey bars at the playground, or jumping double-Dutch rope. Maybe it was playing team sports like softball, basketball, or dodgeball or individual sports like tennis, swimming, or gymnastics. Have you ever put on your favorite music and danced around your room or torn up the dance floor at a fun party? Enjoyed a scenic walk? Had a good full-body stretch after waking from a deep sleep? If you have had any of these experiences, you can channel them to set an intention for the type of movement that you may want to invite into your life.

Experiment with different kinds of movement to see what feels best for you. If you've had negative experiences at the gym in the past, you may want to start with a different setting, perhaps playing with movement at home or out in nature. Movement can be as simple as a stroll around your block. If you want to return to the gym, try different activities than the ones you associate with exercise for weight loss. Perhaps your gym offers water aerobics, dance, stretching, or another class that you haven't tried before. Think about new activities that could be fun to learn. Maybe martial arts like karate, tae kwon do, or capoeira. Games like Ping-Pong and bowling can be a lot of fun. Do you have a trapeze school nearby where you can learn the high ropes? Or perhaps a ninja course or climbing wall? Maybe you like to get out on the water with swimming, kayaking, paddleboarding, or surfing? Or connect with nature while hiking, rock climbing, or biking on local trails? Many yoga studios offer gentle, slow-flow, restorative, or yoga nidra (yogic sleep) classes, which are great opportunities to nurture your body and slow your mind. The possibilities are endless; the key is to think about what is most enjoyable and fun for you that feels yummy in your body.

If you have mobility limitations, these must be considered. Chair yoga, chair qigong, and chair-based strength training are wonderful options for people who have difficulty getting down on the ground for a mat-based class or standing for long periods of time. Many can even be done from a wheelchair. Water-based activities are great because water relieves pressure on the joints, can increase mobility, and can make it easier to move around without pain. If you have mobility limitations or chronic pain, it can be helpful to consult your doctor or work with a physical therapist to integrate movement that eases your pain without exacerbating it.

Leisure Activities and Social Connections

Engaging in enjoyable activities is another important form of self-care. Unfortunately, our capitalist culture is oriented toward productivity, and leisure time can be shunned. Technology has only made this worse, as it has created an expectation that we be available to our jobs seven days a week at all hours. In the US most vacation days go unused, and many of us continue to work even when we are on vacation. This is a recipe for burnout. Even if we are keeping some gas in our tank by engaging in basic self-care, it's hard not to be depleted when we are all work and no fun. A satisfying life is one where we enjoy ourselves. Research suggests that making time for leisure is associated with reduced stress, prevention of depression, increased productivity, increased self-awareness, and increased well-being.[16]

In our busy lives many of us have lost sight of hobbies; the term itself almost seems antiquated. What do you do for fun? If you have a hobby or favorite leisure activity, how often do you do it? Is there a way that you can prioritize leisure time for yourself? Sadly, in our capitalist culture leisure time can be a privilege, afforded to those able to meet their basic needs, including financial security. If it isn't feasible for you to carve out blocks of time for yourself, experiment with taking a few minutes for leisure wherever you can. Perhaps a crossword puzzle on the bus on your way to work, or keeping some art supplies nearby to do a drawing when you find a few spare moments. Joyful movement is one form of leisure activity, but there are many more.

Leisure activities, or hobbies, are unique to each person. One person finds golf deeply fulfilling, while another finds it incredibly boring. Another gets joy from skydiving, while this is someone else's nightmare. Explore what is fun for you. If you don't already have something that you enjoy doing regularly, take a moment and explore what may be appealing to you. It could be anything from knitting to painting, horseback riding, cooking, playing board games, doing jigsaw puzzles, or building model airplanes. If there's something new that you want to learn how to do, consider taking a lesson.

Humans are inherently social creatures; our brains are hardwired that way. While social needs vary from person to person, even the most introverted among us yearns to connect—we all want to be understood. Studies suggest that loneliness has a profound effect on our health.[17] It is estimated that lack of social connections heightens health risks as much as smoking fifteen cigarettes per day or having an alcohol use disorder.[18] Socializing improves mental well-being, confidence and self-esteem, quality of life, immunity and physical health markers, and brain health, while reducing blood pressure and promoting a sense of purpose.[19] Leisure activities can be a great source of social connection. Research suggests that doing an activity with a partner—whether a romantic partner or a friend—can strengthen your relationship, especially if you learn something new together or share a passion.[20] If you don't already have a close social group, you may want to think of new ways to connect with others. It can be hard to make friends as an adult! Joining a book club, ultimate frisbee team, or discussion group on a topic of interest can be a great way to build community. Volunteering, professional organizations, and religious institutions can be other ways of forming social connections and creating a sense of belonging. Check out the fat-positive, body-positive, Health at Every Size, mindful eating, and Intuitive Eating communities online! If social anxiety, depression, or another psychological condition is interfering with your ability to socialize and connect with others, consult with a mental health professional to see if therapy or medications can help.

Pleasure

In 1904 sociologist Max Weber argued that capitalism evolved from Protestantism, a form of Christianity that values consistent diligent hard work ("the Protestant work ethic") and discipline as signs of faith. While we aren't always aware of the religious underpinnings to the capitalistic culture we live in, it influences us nonetheless. We are valued by productivity and accumulation of wealth. An ascetic life, devoid of pleasure, is virtuous. Suffering, self-sacrifice, and martyrdom are idealized, while pleasure is sinful. Using our body as a source of pleasure is especially demonized. "Pleasures of the flesh" and "carnal delights" are religious terms most often associated with sex, but they can refer to any bodily pleasure including eating something delicious, moving our body joyfully, and being touched in pleasurable nonsexual ways like massage, cuddling, hugging, or tickling. Despite these cultural prohibitions, humans are programmed for pleasure, and it is inevitable that we eventually do indulge. When we do, it is often met with guilt, shame, and repentance.

Diet culture, a tool of the capitalist patriarchy, enforces prohibition against pleasure from food (and the fat bodies presumed to result from that pleasure). In this program we've been learning how to question that cultural narrative around food. Now we will also examine the other prohibitions around pleasure in our body and explore unabashedly reconnecting with our body as a source of pleasure.

Many of us were taught that masturbation is something to hide or be ashamed of. If we are religious, we may have been taught that it is a sin, especially combined with "lustful thoughts." We may have learned that it is something that people with penises do but not something that people with vulvas should do. Women are socialized to be dependent on a partner for pleasure, that we should only get off from intercourse, and that our pleasure (or performance of it) is primarily for the benefit of our partner. While most of us masturbate—a 2018 study found that 92 percent of men and 76 percent of women in the US do it—most of us feel it is something to hide.[21] About 55 percent of people say they don't talk about masturbating, and almost 30 percent have lied about it due to embarrassment or fear of being judged. If you have conflicted feelings around sex or experience guilt or shame around pleasuring yourself, please know that sexual pleasure is your birthright, and you can reclaim it. You can use the mindfulness techniques we have been practicing to work with any thoughts of guilt, shame, or criticism that arise while you are connecting to your body for pleasure. When these thoughts come up, use the technique of observing the thoughts, labeling them, centering yourself with your breath, and then compassionately returning your focus to the physical sensations in your body. Trauma can impact sex, and if you are struggling with issues related to sex and trauma, I recommend consulting with a trauma-informed sex therapist, ideally someone practicing from a weight-inclusive perspective.

People who struggle with body image are less likely to masturbate and have enjoyable sexual experiences.[22] It is harder to enjoy sex—either partnered or solo—when you don't feel good about your body. People who have positive body image are more likely to masturbate—or perhaps people who masturbate are more likely to have positive body image. The research isn't clear on which direction this relationship goes, but my guess is that body image and masturbation influence each other. In other words, when we feel good about our body, we are more likely to do things that make our body feel good (like masturbating), and when our body makes us feel good, we are more likely to see that our body *is* good. Will masturbating help you feel better about your body? There's only one way to find out!

Whether or not you already have a regular masturbation practice, I encourage you to approach your body with a beginner's mind and mindfully explore ways to touch yourself for maximal pleasure. Try to set aside some time to really explore your body. If you have never tried it, you may find it useful to examine your genitals with a hand mirror to get a lay of the land. Treat yourself to a solo date night where you start with a relaxing bubble bath, perhaps with some candles or soft music, and build anticipation for the final act of pleasuring yourself. You can rest assured that you'll get lucky at the end of the night! You may want to wear special lingerie or other garments that help you feel sexy. Don't forget the lubrication while you explore. Lube often makes masturbation more pleasurable; one study (albeit one funded by a lubricant manufacturer) found that using lube makes it 50 percent easier to orgasm.[23] Touching yourself without proper lubrication (either from your own body or store-bought) can be painful, especially when using toys.

Research (full disclosure: the study was funded by a sex toy company) suggests that people who use sex toys report being more satisfied with their sex life, including quality and frequency of masturbation.[24] They can be a fun way to add a new element to your routine and experiment with different sensations. Toys are designed for penises and vulvas, as well as nipples, butts, and more. For penises, the most popular toys include masturbation sleeves, rings, plugs, and massagers. For vulvas and vaginas, vibrators are most popular and are designed to be used either internally, externally, or both. Research suggests over 70 percent of people with vulvas need or prefer clitoral stimulation to reach orgasm, so don't forget to give your clitoris some love.[25] Oh, and contrary to what our culture teaches us, pornography isn't just for men! Data from a popular porn site reveals that women made up 32 percent of users in 2019, and another study found that about 31 percent of women say they watch porn about every week.[26] Pornography can include videos, images, erotica (sexy stories that can be either read or listened to), and more. While there is no shortage of online porn sites, it can be more challenging to find quality porn that is produced ethically and doesn't objectify women or fetishize marginalized people. You usually have to pay for the good stuff; consider it an investment in self-care.

There are a ton of benefits to masturbation, including relieving tension, releasing feel-good endorphins, helping you fall asleep, improving self-esteem and body image, relieving menstrual cramps and muscle tension, strengthening pelvic-floor muscles, bettering your mood, improving cognition, strengthening your immune system, increasing sex drive, and helping you feel more empowered sexually. But just like other forms of self-care, masturbation is often couched in terms of health improvements rather than being allowed to stand on its own. We don't need to masturbate because it's good for us. We can just do it because it feels good.

Values

Values are fundamental beliefs that guide our life. They help us decide what is desirable and important to us. They give our life meaning. When we are immersed in diet culture, it sets our values for us and tells us what is most important in our life—shrinking our body. It's all laid out, like a road map to life. When we free ourselves from diet culture, we lose this structure but gain the ability to connect with our core values. When we reflect on our deepest values, most of us realize that our purpose in life is not to become smaller and smaller until we die. We don't want "Had a Great Thigh Gap," "Mastered Atkins," or "Reached Her Goal Weight" written on our tombstones.

How do you want to be remembered? What do you want your life to stand for? What is most meaningful to you? How do you want to spend your time? If you could do anything with your life, without concern for time or money, what would you do? When were you the happiest? Asking yourself these questions can help you identify your core values. Core values may pertain to family, friendship, spirituality, and ways of acting in the world, like honesty, kindness, loyalty, or compassion. Get out a piece of paper and write a list of all the values that come to mind. What are the things in life that are important to you? It may be things like "being a good parent," "adventure," "being a loyal friend," "painting," "engaging in my professional community," "environmental activism," "equity," and so on. Whatever comes to mind, write it down, and give yourself some time to think of as many values as you can. When you are done, go through the list of values and pick the five that are most important to you. These are your core values; they can be used to guide your actions, decisions, and behaviors. Our core values can change over time, so it is important to revisit this list regularly, adding new values and deleting ones that no longer are relevant.

When we don't live in accordance with our values, psychological distress can occur. We may feel like our life is devoid of meaning, that we don't have enough time in the day for the things that are important to us, or that we aren't living our most authentic life. We can feel lost, empty, and depleted. Because of the pressures to keep ourselves as busy as possible, to work as much as possible, to do as much for our children as possible (and make it all social-media-worthy too), many of us are living out of sync with our values and feeling the psychological consequences. Think about how you spend each day. How much time is spent in alignment with your core values? How much time is dedicated to things that are unrelated to your core values? How much time is spent doing things that are in opposition to or contradict your core values? For example, if a core value is family, how much quality time do you spend with your family? If a core value is compassion, do you act in ways that are compassionate toward yourself and others?

Our culture encourages us to live in accordance with the values of capitalism, the patriarchy, diet culture, white supremacy, and other systems of oppression. This makes it hard to always live in accordance with our own values, especially when our values compromise our ability to survive within the cultural framework set for us. For example, it is not uncommon to spend most of our time working, even if this is not a core value. We need to earn money to meet our basic needs. But it may allow us to engage in activities aligned with our core values, like caring for our family or traveling. Nonetheless, living out of sync with our values can lead us to feel unfulfilled. Think of our core values as a compass to guide our life (not a yardstick to beat ourselves up with). Each day we have opportunities to make choices that bring us more in alignment with our values or take us further away. They may be small incremental changes, but they make a difference and shift the path you are on.

Now that our life is dictated less by diet culture, we have more freedom to live in ways that are most meaningful and fulfilling. We can direct more of our energy to what's most important to us. Whether that is spending time with family, creating beauty in the world, or engaging in activism, we can commit ourselves most fully when we aren't dedicating our life to the demands of diet culture. What are you going to do with all the time, energy, and money that you reclaim from dieting? This isn't the end; it is just the beginning. My hope is that this book has set you on a path toward being more accepting and compassionate with your body, more present in your life, embracing the joy of eating, finding pleasure in your body, and living a meaningful, valuable, and satisfying life. Now it's time to go out in the world and reclaim all that dieting has stolen from you, to capture the pleasure that is rightfully yours, and take up the space that you deserve!

TAKE-ACTION ACTIVITIES

Find your needs

Make a list of your basic self-care needs. Consider food, drink, sleep, hygiene, health, and safety. How many of these basic needs are being met? What can you do to better meet these needs?

Find a way to move

Pick a type of movement that seems enjoyable. It could be walking, dancing, hiking, tennis, dodgeball, tai chi, stretching, yoga ... the possibilities are endless. Set aside time this week to engage in this activity. If you try something and you don't like it, set aside another time to try a different activity, and keep testing out different ones until you find something you enjoy. Remember, it doesn't need to be anything time-consuming or fancy; a walk around your block or stretching at home are great options. Try to keep a compassionate, nonjudgmental, non-goal-oriented approach to the movement, staying fully present with yourself and attuned to your body.

Find your pleasure

Identify ways to cultivate pleasure in your body, and set a date to engage in at least one of these activities this week. Feel free to think outside of the box, but if you are feeling stuck, here are some ideas. Put your pleasure date on your calendar and don't let anything get in the way!

- Mindfully and lovingly apply lotion to your body. You can use a scented lotion (if you don't have a sensitivity to perfumes) and use your mindfulness skills to fully take in the scent of the lotion and all the sensations of rubbing the lotion into your skin. You can even experiment with giving yourself a mini-massage while you are applying the lotion.

- Take a bubble bath. Notice the sensations of your skin in the warm water, the feelings of your muscles relaxing in the warmth of the bath, the texture and sensations of the bubbles, as well as any scents that may be present.

- Get a massage. If a professional massage isn't in your budget, you can trade massages with a partner. Allow yourself to fully enjoy the pleasure of someone else touching and massaging your body.

- Mindfully eat something delicious. Allow yourself to mindfully eat something that you really enjoy, and savor every bite!

- Masturbate. Bring a "beginner's mind" to the experience and allow yourself the time to relish in your body. You may set the mood for yourself with candles, music, lingerie, and anything else that helps you feel sexy. Lubricant, sex toys, and pornography can be fun tools in self-pleasuring.

Find your fun

What are your hobbies or favorite leisure activities? Are you satisfying your leisure needs? You may find that you need to regularly set aside time for recreation. Look at your calendar and plan time to engage in at least one fun leisure activity this week.

Find your connections

How do you connect with others? Where is your community? Do you feel your social needs are being satisfied? What obstacles or barriers do you face in meeting your social needs? Think about ways to best meet these needs. Is there a group you could join, a class you would like to take, or a cultural or religious institution you want to get more involved with? Plan at least one thing you can do this week to care for your social needs.

Find your values

Identify your core values. Answer the following questions in your journal:

- What brings meaning to your life?
- What do you stand for? What are your principles?
- What roles are important to you?
- What ignites your passion?
- What makes you excited to wake up in the morning?
- What kind of a life do you want to live?
- If you could do anything with your life, without concern for time or money, what would you be doing?
- When were you the happiest?
- What would you want people to say at your funeral about your life and what kind of person you were?

After answering those questions, write down as many of your values as you can. Values can be things like "honesty," "compassion," "being a loyal friend," "being a good parent," "creating art," or "social justice activism." Spend at least ten minutes pouring out all your values you can think of. Then go through the list and identify the five values that are most important to you. These are your core values. How can you live your life most in accordance with your core values? Is your relationship with food and your body in alignment with your core values? Does the way that you spend your time and resources align with your core values? Use these core values as a compass to guide decisions, actions, and behaviors in your life.

Reflect on all you've done and all you want to do

Now that you have completed this program, take some time to reflect on your experience in your journal. What has changed since you started this book? Do you approach food differently? Are you more aware of your body's internal GPS signals like hunger, fullness, taste, cravings, and your body's reactions to different foods? Have you become more compassionate with yourself? More present in your life? More accepting of your body? Remember, this program is intended to serve as a stepping-stone to set you on a different path in your relationship with food and body image, but it's not the end of your journey. What do you want to work on next?

Continue meditating

I hope that this program has helped you build a regular meditation practice, one that has become a valuable part of your daily routine, and one that you want to sustain long after the end of this book. Continue meditating daily either using the three-, five-, or fifteen-minute meditation available at www.drconason.com/diet-free-revolution/ or setting a timer and leading yourself through the meditation practice. If you are consistently meditating for fifteen minutes each day, experiment with increasing your practice to twenty minutes per day. Feel free to explore the different mindfulness meditation resources available online (including apps, guided meditations, mindfulness courses, and even online meditation retreats), at bookstores, and locally if you live near a mindfulness meditation center or a yoga studio that offers meditation classes.

Appendix

Meditations and Mindful Eating Practice

Breathing Mindful Breaths, p. 84

Bringing full awareness and attention to our breath is the foundation of our practice. But breath isn't the point of meditation—breath is a tool to observe the activity of the mind. Learn to use your breath to focus your mind.

Meditate Daily with Five Minutes of Mindful Breath, p. 88

Find a comfortable location, then listen to a guided meditation to begin your own mindfulness meditation practice. For best results, pick a time when this five-minute break can consistently fit into your usual schedule.

Taking a Mindful Pause, and Integrating It into Your Daily Routine, p. 86 and p. 88

Through five simple steps, the mindful pause helps you tune in to your body's hunger, fullness, cravings, and more. Set an alert on your phone to check in with yourself at random points during your day. And prior to eating, take a mindful pause to check in with your body and become present with your food.

Apply Your Mindfulness Skills to Your Eating, p. 89

This practice engages all your senses to help you become fully present with the food you're eating. By taking a moment to notice the appearance, feel, smell, taste, and texture of your food—and your body's reactions to it—you will build your mindfulness and bodily awareness.

Be Self-Compassionate, p. 107

Follow a guided audio meditation on self-compassion. Try a body gratitude exercise that helped improve people's body image and reduce their internalized weight bias in a research study. And set your intention to do at least one kind act for yourself this week.

Practice Quieting Your Inner Critic, p. 107

By acknowledging instead of trying to ignore (or obey) an inner critic, you can limit its ability to distract you. When you notice your inner critic speaking up, label it, shift your awareness to the present moment, and then move forward with compassion.

Understand Your Hunger Better, p. 127

Fill out the Hunger Scale with your own physical symptoms of feeling hungry; everyone's are different. Identify the sensations that accompany your different levels of hunger. Take a mindful pause for hunger before you eat, and eat a mindful meal focusing on your hunger awareness.

Scan Your Whole Body for Cues, p. 128

Try the body scan meditation by following a guided audio recording. From the tips of your toes to the top of your head, notice all the bodily sensations that are present.

Meditate a Bit Longer, p. 141

Try increasing your daily meditation practice to ten or fifteen minutes. Still simply focus on your breath, notice when your mind wanders, and gently bring your awareness back to your breath. Follow our guided audio meditation, or experiment with ones available online (just make sure they're *mindfulness* meditations—other types don't foster the skills we're building).

Notice Your Fullness Mindfully, p. 143

As you're eating a meal, pay close attention to how your fullness changes. Can you identify the first signs of fullness emerging? How a 1 feels different from a 2 on the Fullness Scale? Where's your comfortable point to stop eating?

Mindful Eating with Nuts, p. 144

First take a mindful pause to check in with yourself. Then notice the details of the nuts in front of you—their shape, feel, color, aroma, and taste. (If you are allergic or if your body doesn't respond well to this food, substitute a similar dense snack for this exercise.) After eating one nut, identify where you are on the Hunger and Fullness Scales. As you mindfully eat more nuts one by one, can you tell when those numbers change?

Be Taste-Aware with Chocolate, p. 161

After taking a mindful pause, closely observe some of your favorite chocolate—and your own thoughts or feelings about it. (If you are allergic or really dislike chocolate, feel free to substitute something similar that works better for you.) Mindfully eat a piece, and give yourself a rating on the Taste Enjoyment Scale. Repeat the process with another piece. Did you perceive any changes in taste from the first to second piece of chocolate?

Be Taste-Aware through a Meal, p. 162

Eat a mindful meal focusing on awareness of taste and how taste changes as you eat. Rate your first bite on the Taste Enjoyment Scale, then continue making ratings for each bite. Checking in with yourself and giving ratings on the scale can help you decide if you're still enjoying the food.

Have a Mindful Meal Out, p. 185

At a restaurant, take a mindful pause for hunger and fullness. Leisurely peruse the menu items, including dishes that don't usually appeal, and identify what you're in the mood for. Take another mindful pause when your food arrives. Rate your first bite on the Taste Enjoyment Scale. Keep eating mindfully, and note the point where you feel satisfied. Do any feelings arise?

Practice Mindful Cooking, p. 186

Bring your mindfulness skills to all aspects of making a meal. Notice the appearance, textures, and smells of ingredients, the sounds of preparation and cooking. Think about how all the ingredients combined to make this dish. Can you taste each one? Lead yourself through eating the dish mindfully.

Eat Mindfully from Many Choices, p. 186

At a buffet or family-style meal, take a moment to check out all options before putting anything on your plate. What seems appealing? Want to try something new? Mindfully eat what you've selected, and notice how your body reacts to the different foods. Check in with your hunger, fullness, and taste. Repeat the whole process until you feel satisfied.

Explore Abundance, p. 187

If you struggle with feeling out of control around a certain food, try welcoming it in abundance. When you don't feel this food is scarce, it has less influence on you. Stock your pantry with plenty of it. If you eat "too much" and don't feel well, treat your body and mind with compassion—and then buy more.

Gratitude Meditation for Emotional Eating, p. 206

Think about a time you ate emotionally; try to recall how you were feeling, what emotions triggered you to eat, and how you acted toward yourself afterward. After some mindful breathing, envision the emotional eating experience again, but this time bathe yourself in self-compassion, love, and kindness—can you thank food for helping you get through that difficult time?

Mindful Pause for Emotions, p. 207

In a mindful meditation, expand your awareness to any emotions you can notice. Where in your body do you feel them? Do you have thoughts or feelings about them? Can you label them? Be patient and gentle with yourself—identifying feelings can be hard. Recognizing one, even if you can't name it, is an important step in itself.

Practice These Three Steps When You Have the Urge to Eat Emotionally, p. 208

Identify hunger (where are you on the scale? Eat if you are hungry), then identify your emotions (take a mindful pause, and label what you can), then meet your emotional needs (care for yourself in the moment). Make a choice that feels compassionate, nurturing, and in tune with your present feelings. Whatever you choose—contacting a friend, taking a nap, eating—do it without judgment.

Notes

Introduction

1 "How to Become a WW Lifetime Member," WW International, Inc., February 7, 2020, www.weightwatchers.com/us/blog/weight-loss/lifetime-membership.

2 "WW Announces Fourth Quarter and Full Year 2019 Results and Provides Full Year 2020 Guidance," WW International, Inc., February 25, 2020, www.globenewswire .com/news-release/2020/02/25/1990458/0/en/WW-Announces-Fourth-Quarter-and -Full-Year-2019-Results-and-Provides-Full-Year-2020-Guidance.html.

3 C. B. Martin, K. A. Herrick, N. Sarafrazi, and C. L. Ogden, "Attempts to Lose Weight among Adults in the United States, 2013–2016," NCHS Data Brief, no. 313, National Center for Health Statistics, 2018, www.cdc.gov/nchs/products/databriefs /db313.htm.

4 Research and Markets, "United States Weight Loss and Diet Control Market Report 2019: Value and Growth Rates of All Major Weight Loss Segments—Early 1980s to 2018, 2019 and 2023 Forecasts," February 25, 2019, www.globenewswire.com /news-release/2019/02/25/1741719/0/en/United-States-Weight-Loss-Diet-Control -Market-Report-2019-Value-Growth-Rates-of-All-Major-Weight-Loss-Segments -Early-1980s-to-2018-2019-and-2023-Forecasts.html.

5 "Statistics and Facts," Global Wellness Institute, September 21, 2020, www .globalwellnessinstitute.org/press-room/statistics-and-facts/.

6 "100 Million Dieters, $20 Billion: The Weight-Loss Industry by the Numbers," ABC News, May 7, 2012, https://abcnews.go.com/Health/100-million-dieters-20-billion -weight-loss-industry/story?id=16297197.

7 Love Fresh Berries, "January Fad Diets" (press release), 2019.

8 Naomi Wolf, *The Beauty Myth: How Images of Beauty Are Used against Women* (London: Vintage, 1991), 187.

9 N. Graf, A. Brown, and E. Patten, "The Narrowing, but Persistent, Gender Gap in Pay," Pew Research Center, August 14, 2020, www.pewresearch.org/fact-tank /2019/03/22/gender-pay-gap-facts/; "Black Women Aren't Paid Fairly—and That Hits Harder in an Economic Crisis," Lean In, n.d., retrieved October 15, 2020, www.leanin.org/data-about-the-gender-pay-gap-for-black-women.

10 Alisha Coleman-Jensen, Matthew P. Rabbitt, Christian A. Gregory, and Anita Singh, "Household Food Security in the United States in 2018," no. ERR-270, 2019, Economic Research Service, US Department of Agriculture, www.ers.usda.gov /publications/pub-details/?pubid=94848.

11 C. D. Runfola, A. Von Holle, S. E. Trace, K. A. Brownley, S. M. Hofmeier, D. A. Gagne, and C. M. Bulik, "Body Dissatisfaction in Women across the Lifespan: Results of the UNC-*SELF* and Gender and Body Image (GABI) Studies," *European Eating Disorders Review* 21, no. 1 (2013): 52–59, www.doi.org/10.1002/erv.2201; D. A. Frederick, A. M. Jafary, K. Gruys, and E. A. Daniels, "Surveys and the Epidemiology of Body Image Dissatisfaction," in *Encyclopedia of Body Image and Human Appearance*, ed. Thomas F. Cash, (Amsterdam: Academic Press, 2012) 766–74.

Chapter 1

1 Raj Chetty, Michael Stepner, Sarah Abraham, Shelby Lin, Benjamin Scuderi, Nicholas Turner, Augustin Bergeron, and David Cutler, "The Association between Income and Life Expectancy in the United States, 2001–2014," *JAMA* 315, no. 16 (2016): 1750–66, www.doi.org/10.1001/jama.2016.4226.

2 Cynthia L. Ogden, Tala H. Fakhouri, Margaret D. Carroll, Craig M. Hales, Cheryl D. Fryar, Xianfen Li, and David S. Freedman, "Prevalence of Obesity among Adults, by Household Income and Education—United States, 2011–2014," *Morbidity and Mortality Weekly Report* 66, no. 50 (2017): 1369–73, www.doi.org/10.15585/mmwr .mm6650a1; James A. Levine, "Poverty and Obesity in the US," *Diabetes* 60, no. 11 (November 2011): 2667–68, www.doi.org/10.2337/db11-1118; Robert Rogers, Taylor F. Eagle, Anne Sheetz, Alan Woodward, Robert Leibowitz, MinKyoung Song, Rachel Sylvester, Nicole Corriveau, Eva Kline-Rogers, Qingmei Jiang, Elizabeth A. Jackson, and Kim A. Eagle, "The Relationship between Childhood Obesity, Low Socioeconomic Status, and Race/Ethnicity: Lessons from Massachusetts," *Childhood Obesity* 11, no. 6 (December 2015): 691–95, www.doi.org/10.1089/chi.2015.0029.

3 A. Stunkard and M. McLaren-Hume, "The Results of Treatment for Obesity: A Review of the Literature and Report of a Series," *Archives of Internal Medicine* 103, no. 1 (1959): 79–85.

4 R. R. Wing and S. Phelan, "Long-Term Weight Loss Maintenance," *American Journal of Clinical Nutrition* 82, no. 1 (2005): 222S–225S, www.doi.org/10.1093 /ajcn/82.1.222S; S. Sarlio-Lähteenkorva, A. Rissanen, and J. Kaprio, "A Descriptive Study of Weight Loss Maintenance: 6 and 15 Year Follow-Up of Initially Overweight

Adults," *International Journal of Obesity and Related Metabolic Disorders* 24, no. 1 (January 2000): 116–25, www.doi.org/10.1038/sj.ijo.0801094.

5   T. Mann, A. J. Tomiyama, E. Westling, A.-M. Lew, B. Samuels, and J. Chatman, "Medicare's Search for Effective Obesity Treatments: Diets Are Not the Answer," *American Psychologist* 62, no. 3 (2007): 220–33.

6   The Look AHEAD Research Group, "Cardiovascular Effects of Intensive Lifestyle Intervention in Type 2 Diabetes," *New England Journal of Medicine* 369 (2013): 145–54, www.doi.org/10.1056/NEJMoa1212914.

7   The Look AHEAD Research Group, "The Look AHEAD Study: A Description of the Lifestyle Intervention and the Evidence Supporting It," *Obesity* 14, no. 5 (2006): 737–52, www.doi.org/10.1038/oby.2006.84.

8   The Look AHEAD Research Group, "Eight-Year Weight Losses with an Intensive Lifestyle Intervention: The Look AHEAD Study," *Obesity* 22, no. 1 (2014): 5–13, www.doi.org/10.1002/oby.20662; The Look AHEAD Research Group, "Cardiovascular Effects of Intensive Lifestyle Intervention in Type 2 Diabetes," *New England Journal of Medicine* 369 (2013): 145–54, www.doi.org/10.1056/NEJMoa1212914; X. Pi-Sunyer, "The Look AHEAD Trial: A Review and Discussion of Its Outcomes," *Current Nutrition Reports* 3, no. 4 (2014): 387–91, www.doi.org/10.1007/s13668 -014-0099-x; M. G. Salvia, "The Look AHEAD Trial: Translating Lessons Learned into Clinical Practice and Further Study," *Diabetes Spectrum* 30, no. 3 (August 2017): 166–70, www.doi.org/10.2337/ds17-0016.

9   R. Wing and J. Hill, "The National Weight Control Registry," n.d., retrieved October 8, 2020, www.nwcr.ws/default.htm.

10   R. Chastain, "Do 95% of Dieters Really Fail?" *Dances with Fat* (blog), July 11, 2012, www.danceswithfat.org/2011/06/28/do-95-of-dieters-really-fail/.

11   L. M. Gianini, B. T. Walsh, J. Steinglass, and L. Mayer, "Long-Term Weight Loss Maintenance in Obesity: Possible Insights from Anorexia Nervosa?" *International Journal of Eating Disorders* 50, no. 4 (2017): 341–42, www.doi.org/10.1002/eat.22685.

12   A. Keys, J. Brozek, A. Henshel, O. Mickelson, and H. L. Taylor, *The Biology of Human Starvation*, vols. 1–2 (Minneapolis: University of Minnesota Press, 1950).

13   D. Baker and N. Keramidas, "The Psychology of Hunger," *Monitor on Psychology* 44, no. 9 (October 2013), www.apa.org/monitor/2013/10/hunger.

14   C. P. Herman and D. Mack, "Restrained and Unrestrained Eating," *Journal of Personality* 43 (1975): 647–60.

15   J. S. Coelho, J. Polivy, and C. P. Herman, "Selective Carbohydrate or Protein Restriction: Effects on Subsequent Food Intake and Cravings," *Appetite* 47 (2006): 352–60, www.doi.org/10.1016/j.appet.2006.05.015.

16   R. L. Leibel, M. Rosenbaum, and J. Hirsch, "Changes in Energy Expenditure Resulting from Altered Body Weight, *New England Journal of Medicine* 332, no. 10 (March 9, 1995): 621–28, www.doi.org/10.1056/NEJM199503093321001.

17   W. Gibbs, "Interview with Rudolph L. Leibel," *Scientific American*, August 8, 1996, www.scientificamerican.com/article/interview-with-rudolph-l/.

18   E. Fothergill, J. Guo, L. Howard, J. C. Kerns, N. D. Knuth, R. Brychta, K. Y. Chen, M. C. Skarulis, M. Walter, P. J. Walter, and K. D. Hall, "Persistent Metabolic Adaptation 6 Years after 'The Biggest Loser' Competition," *Obesity* 24, no. 8 (August 2016): 1612–19, www.doi.org/10.1002/oby.21538.

19   S. E. Domoff, N. G. Hinman, A. M. Koball, A. Storfer-Isser, V. L. Carhart, K. D. Baik, and R. A. Carel, "The Effects of Reality Television on Weight Bias: An Examination of 'The Biggest Loser,'" *Obesity* 20, no. 5 (May 2012): 993–98, www.doi.org/10.1038/oby.2011.378.

20   P. Sumithran, L. A. Prendergast, E. Delbridge, K. Purcell, A. Shulkes, A. Kriketos, and J. Proietto, "Long-Term Persistence of Hormonal Adaptations to Weight Loss," *New England Journal of Medicine* 365, no. 17 (October 27, 2011): 1597–604, www.doi.org/10.1056/NEJMoa1105816.

21   A. J. Hill, "The Psychology of Food Craving," *Proceedings of the Nutrition Society* 66, no. 2 (2007): 277–85, www.doi.org/10.1017/S0029665107005502.

22   Rudolph Leibel and Jules Hirsch, interview by Charlie Rose, *Charlie Rose*, March 9, 1995, www.charlierose.com/videos/4861.

Chapter 2

1   "Rheumatoid Arthritis," Mayo Clinic, March 1, 2019, www.mayoclinic.org/diseases-conditions/rheumatoid-arthritis/diagnosis-treatment/drc-20353653.

2   A. Kassam, "Canadian Woman Uses Own Obituary to Rail against Fat-Shaming," *Guardian*, July 30, 2018, www.theguardian.com/world/2018/jul/30/canada-ellen-maud-bennett-obituary-fat-shaming.

3   R. M. Puhl and K. D. Brownell, "Confronting and Coping with Weight Stigma: An Investigation of Overweight and Obese Adults," *Obesity* 14, no. 10 (2006): 1802–15, www.doi.org/10.1038/oby.2006.208.

4   R. M. Puhl and C. A. Heuer, "The Stigma of Obesity: A Review and Update," *Obesity* 17, no. 5 (2009): 941–64, www.doi.org/10.1038/oby.2008.636; G. D. Foster, T. A. Wadden, A. P. Makris, D. Davidson, R. S. Sanderson, D. B. Allison, and A. Kessler, "Primary Care Physicians' Attitudes about Obesity and Its Treatment," *Obesity Resources* 11, no. 10 (2003): 1168–77, www.doi.org/10.1038/oby.2003.161; A. Bocquier, P. Verger, A. Basdevant, G. Andreotti, J. Baretge, P. Villani, and A. Paraponaris, "Overweight and Obesity: Knowledge, Attitudes, and Practices of General Practitioners in France," *Obesity Resources* 13, no. 4 (2005): 787–95, www.doi.org/10.1038/oby.2005.89.

5   R. M. Puhl and C. A. Heuer, "The Stigma of Obesity: A Review and Update," *Obesity* 17, no. 5 (2009): 941–64, www.doi.org/10.1038/oby.2008.636.

6   G. Geller and P. Watkins, "Addressing Medical Students' Negative Bias toward Patients with Obesity through Ethics Education," *AMA Journal of Ethics* 20, no. 10 (2018): E948–59, www.doi.org/10.1001/amajethics.2018.948.

7   R. L. Pearl, D. Argueso, and T. A. Wadden, "Effects of Medical Trainees' Weight-Loss History on Perceptions of Patients with Obesity," *Medical Education* 51, no. 8 (August 2017): 802–11, www.doi.org/10.1111/medu.13275.

8   D. Wear, J. M. Aultman, J. D. Varley, and J. Zarconi, "Making Fun of Patients: Medical Students' Perceptions and Use of Derogatory and Cynical Humor in Clinical Settings," *Academic Medicine* 81, no. 5 (2006): 454–62, www.doi.org/10.1097/01 .ACM.0000222277.21200.a1.

9   A. Bocquier, P. Verger, A. Basdevant, G. Andreotti, J. Baretge, P. Villani, and A. Paraponaris, "Overweight and Obesity: Knowledge, Attitudes, and Practices of General Practitioners in France," *Obesity Resources* 13, no. 4 (2005): 787–95, www.doi.org /10.1038/oby.2005.89.

10 S. M. Phelan, D. J. Burgess, M. W. Yeazel, W. L. Hellerstedt, J. M. Griffin, and M. van Ryn, "Impact of Weight Bias and Stigma on Quality of Care and Outcomes for Patients with Obesity," *Obesity Reviews* 16, no. 4 (April 2015): 319–26, www.doi.org /10.1111/obr.12266.

11 R. M. Puhl and C. A. Heuer, "The Stigma of Obesity: A Review and Update," *Obesity* 17, no. 5 (2009): 941–64, www.doi.org/10.1038/oby.2008.636.

12 C. H. Adams, N. J. Smith, D. C. Wilbur, and K. E. Grady, "The Relationship of Obesity to the Frequency of Pelvic Examinations: Do Physician and Patient Attitudes Make a Difference?" *Women and Health* 20, no. 2 (1993): 45–57, www.doi.org /10.1300/j013v20n02_04.

13 S. M. Phelan, D. J. Burgess, M. W. Yeazel, W. L. Hellerstedt, J. M. Griffin, and M. van Ryn, "Impact of Weight Bias and Stigma on Quality of Care and Outcomes for Patients with Obesity," *Obesity Reviews* 16, no. 4 (April 2015): 319–26, www.doi.org /10.1111/obr.12266.

14 "What Is Patient-Centered Care?" *NEJM Catalyst*, January 2017, https://catalyst .nejm.org/doi/full/10.1056/CAT.17.0559.

15 M. H. Kramer, W. Bauer, D. Dicker, M. Durusu-Tanriover, F. Ferreira, S. P. Rigby, X. Roux, P. M. Schumm-Draeger, F. Weidanz, J. H. van Hulsteijn, "The Changing Face of Internal Medicine: Patient Centred Care," *European Journal of Internal Medicine* 25, no. 2 (February 2014): 125–27, www.doi.org/10.1016/j.ejim .2013.11.013.

16 S. M. Phelan, D. J. Burgess, M. W. Yeazel, W. L. Hellerstedt, J. M. Griffin, and M. van Ryn, "Impact of Weight Bias and Stigma on Quality of Care and Outcomes for Patients with Obesity," *Obesity Reviews* 16, no. 4 (April 2015): 319–26, www .doi.org/10.1111/obr.12266; R. M. Puhl and C. A. Heuer, "The Stigma of Obesity: A Review and Update," *Obesity* 17, no. 5 (2009): 941–64, www.doi.org/10.1038 /oby.2008.636.

17 N. K. Amy, A. Aalborg, P. Lyons, and L. Keranen, "Barriers to Routine Gynecological Cancer Screening for White and African-American Obese Women," *International*

Journal of Obesity 30, no. 1 (January 2006): 147–55, www.doi.org/10.1038/sj.ijo.0803105.

18 C. A. A. Drury and M. Louis, "Exploring the Association between Body Weight, Stigma of Obesity, and Health Care Avoidance," *Journal of the American Academy of Nurse Practitioners* 14, no. 12 (2002): 554–60, www.doi.org/10.1111/j.1745-7599.2002.tb00089.x.

19 A. J. Tomiyama, D. Carr, E. M. Granberg, B. Major, E. Robinson, A. R. Sutin, and A. Brewis, "How and Why Weight Stigma Drives the Obesity 'Epidemic' and Harms Health," *BMC Medicine* 16, no. 1 (2018): 123, www.doi.org/10.1186/s12916-018-1116-5.

20 "Crunching Numbers: What Cancer Screening Statistics Really Tell Us," National Cancer Institute, July 2018, www.cancer.gov/about-cancer/screening/research/what-screening-statistics-mean.

21 R. M. Puhl and C. A. Heuer, "The Stigma of Obesity: A Review and Update," *Obesity* 17, no. 5 (2009): 941–64, www.doi.org/10.1038/oby.2008.636.

22 K. E. Friedman, S. K. Reichmann, P. R. Costanzo, A. Zelli, J. A. Ashmore, and G. J. Musante, "Weight Stigmatization and Ideological Beliefs: Relation to Psychological Functioning in Obese Adults," *Obesity Research* 13, no. 5 (May 2005): 907–16, www.doi.org/10.1038/oby.2005.105.

23 R. M. Puhl and C. A. Heuer, "The Stigma of Obesity: A Review and Update," *Obesity* 17, no. 5 (2009): 941–64, www.doi.org/10.1038/oby.2008.636.

24 R. Puhl, S. Telke, N. Larson, M. Eisenberg, and D. Neumark-Stzainer, "Experiences of Weight Stigma and Links with Self-Compassion among a Population-Based Sample of Young Adults from Diverse Ethnic/Racial and Socio-economic Backgrounds," *Journal of Psychosomatic Research* 134 (2020): 110134, www.doi.org/10.1016/j.jpsychores.2020.110134.

25 R. Pearl, M. Himmelstein, R. Puhl, T. Wadden, A. Wojtanowski, and G. Foster, "Weight Bias Internalization in a Commercial Weight Management Sample: Prevalence and Correlates," *Obesity Science and Practice* 5, no. 4 (2019): 342–53, www.doi.org/10.1002/osp4.354.

26 R. L. Pearl, T. A. Wadden, C. M. Hopkins, J. A. Shaw, M. R. Hayes, Z. M. Bakizada, N. Alfaris, A. M. Chao, E. Pinkasavage, R. I. Berkowitz, and N. Alamuddin, "Association between Weight Bias Internalization and Metabolic Syndrome among Treatment-Seeking Individuals with Obesity," *Obesity* 25, no. 2 (2017): 317–22, www.doi.org/10.1002/oby.21716.

27 R. Pearl, M. Himmelstein, R. Puhl, T. Wadden, A. Wojtanowski, and G. Foster, "Weight Bias Internalization in a Commercial Weight Management Sample: Prevalence and Correlates," *Obesity Science and Practice* 5, no. 4 (2019): 342–53, www.doi.org/10.1002/osp4.354.

28 R. M. Puhl and C. A. Heuer, "The Stigma of Obesity: A Review and Update," *Obesity* 17, no. 5 (2009): 941–64, www.doi.org/10.1038/oby.2008.636.

29 R. M. Puhl and C. A. Heuer, "The Stigma of Obesity: A Review and Update," *Obesity* 17, no. 5 (2009): 941–64, www.doi.org/10.1038/oby.2008.636.

30 Y. K. Wu and D. C. Berry, "Impact of Weight Stigma on Physiological and Psychological Health Outcomes for Overweight and Obese Adults: A Systematic Review," *Journal of Advanced Nursing* 74, no. 5 (May 2018): 1030–42, www.doi.org/10.1111/jan.13511; R. L. Pearl, T. A. Wadden, C. M. Hopkins, J. A. Shaw, M. R. Hayes, Z. M. Bakizada, N. Alfaris, A. M. Chao, E. Pinkasavage, R. I. Berkowitz, and N. Alamuddin, "Association between Weight Bias Internalization and Metabolic Syndrome among Treatment-Seeking Individuals with Obesity," *Obesity* 25, no. 2 (2017): 317–22, www.doi.org/10.1002/oby.21716.

31 R. Chetty, M. Stepner, S. Abraham, S. Lin, B. Scuderi, N. Turner, A. Bergeron, and D. Cutler, "The Association between Income and Life Expectancy in the United States, 2001–2014," *JAMA* 315, no. 16 (2016): 1750–66, www.doi.org/10.1001/jama.2016.4226.

32 J.-P. Montani, Y. Schutz, and A. G. Dulloo, "Dieting and Weight Cycling as Risk Factors for Cardiometabolic Diseases: Who Is Really at Risk?" *Obesity Reviews* 16, no. S1 (2015): 7–18, www.doi.org/10.1111/obr.12251; J.-P. Montani, A. K. Viecelli, A. Prévot, and A. G. Dulloo, "Weight Cycling during Growth and Beyond as a Risk Factor for Later Cardiovascular Diseases: The 'Repeated Overshoot' Theory," *International Journal of Obesity* 30, no. S4 (2006): S58–66, www.doi.org/10.1038/sj.ijo.0803520.

33 R. A. Murphy, K. V. Patel, S. B. Kritchevsky, D. K. Houston, A. B. Newman, A. Koster, E. M. Simonsick, F. A. Tylvasky, P. M. Cawthon, and T. B. Harris, "Weight Change, Body Composition, and Risk of Mobility Disability and Mortality in Older Adults: A Population-Based Cohort Study," *Journal of the American Geriatrics Society* 62, no. 8 (2014): 1476–83, www.doi.org/10.1111/jgs.12954.

34 Tae Jung Oh, Jae Hoon Moon, Sung Hee Choi, Soo Lim, Kyong Soo Park, Nam H. Cho, and Hak Chul Jang, "Body-Weight Fluctuation and Incident Diabetes Mellitus, Cardiovascular Disease, and Mortality: A 16-Year Prospective Cohort Study," *Journal of Clinical Endocrinology and Metabolism* 104, no. 3 (March 2019): 639–46, www.doi.org/10.1210/jc.2018-01239.

35 K. D. Brownell and J. Rodin, "Medical, Metabolic, and Psychological Effects of Weight Cycling," *Archives of Internal Medicine* 154, no. 12 (June 27, 1994): 1325–30.

36 K. Strohacker and B. K. McFarlin, "Influence of Obesity, Physical Inactivity, and Weight Cycling on Chronic Inflammation," *Frontiers in Bioscience* 2 (January 2010): 98–104, www.doi.org/10.2741/e70; K. Strohacker, K. C. Carpenter, and B. K. McFarlin, "Consequences of Weight Cycling: An Increase in Disease Risk?" *International Journal of Exercise Science* 2, no. 3 (2009): 191–201.

37 Sabrina Strings, *Fearing the Black Body: The Racial Origins of Fat Phobia* (New York: New York University Press, 2019).

38 "Body Mass Index: Considerations for Practitioners," Centers for Disease Control and Prevention, n.d., retrieved December 11, 2020, www.cdc.gov/obesity/downloads /bmiforpactitioners.pdf.

39 F. Q. Nuttall, "Body Mass Index: Obesity, BMI, and Health: A Critical Review," *Nutrition Today* 50, no. 3 (2015): 117–128, www.doi.org/10.1097/NT.0000000000000092; R. Moynihan, "Obesity Task Force Linked to WHO Takes 'Millions' from Drug Firms," *BMJ* 332 (2006): 1412, www.doi.org/10.1136/bmj.332.7555.1412-a.

40 Kiera Butler, "Why BMI Is a Big Fat Scam," *Mother Jones*, August 25, 2014, www.motherjones.com/politics/2014/08/why-bmi-big-fat-scam/.

41 American Medical Association Council on Science and Public Health, *Proceedings of the 2013 Annual Meeting of the American Medical Association House of Delegates, Reports of the Council on Science and Public Health*, 2013, 335–43, www.ama-assn.org /sites/ama-assn.org/files/corp/media-browser/public/hod/a13-csaph-reports_0.pdf.

42 A. Pollack, "AMA Recognizes Obesity as a Disease," *New York Times*, June 18, 2013, http://nyti.ms/1Guko03.

43 "Recognition of Obesity as a Disease—Resolution: 420," American Medical Association House of Delegates, May 16, 2013, http://media.npr.org/documents/2013/jun /ama-resolution-obesity.pdf.

44 Caroline M. Apovian, Louis J. Aronne, Daniel H. Bessesen, Marie E. McDonnell, M. Hassan Murad, Uberto Pagotto, Donna H. Ryan, and Christopher D. Still, "Pharmacological Management of Obesity: An Endocrine Society Clinical Practice Guideline," *Journal of Clinical Endocrinology and Metabolism* 100, no. 2 (February 1, 2015): 342–62, www.doi.org/10.1210/jc.2014-3415.

45 "Caroline Apovian MD, FACP, FACN," EndocrineWeb, n.d., retrieved November 15, 2020, www.endocrineweb.com/author/17628/apovian.

46 "OAC Chairman's Council," Obesity Action Coalition, n.d., retrieved November 15, 2020, www.obesityaction.org/community/donate/ways-to-give/oac-chairmans-council/; "Clients," Potomac Currents, n.d., retrieved February 16, 2021, www.potomaccurrents .com/clients.html.

47 Kay-Tee Khaw, Nicholas Wareham, Sheila Bingham, Ailsa Welch, Robert Luben, and Nicholas Day, "Combined Impact of Health Behaviours and Mortality in Men and Women: The EPIC-Norfolk Prospective Population Study," *PLoS Medicine* 5, no. 1 (2008): e12, www.doi.org/10.1371/journal.pmed.0050012.

48 E. Matheson, D. King, and C. Everett, "Healthy Lifestyle Habits and Mortality in Overweight and Obese Individuals," *Journal of the American Board of Family Medicine* 25, no. 1 (2012): 9–15, www.doi.org/10.3122/jabfm.2012.01.110164.

49 V. W. Barry, M. Baruth, M. W. Beets, J. L. Durstine, J. Liu, and S. N. Blair, "Fitness vs. Fatness on All-Cause Mortality: A Meta-Analysis," *Progress in Cardiovascular Diseases* 56, no. 4 (January–February 2014): 382–90, www.doi.org/10.1016/j.pcad.2013.09.002.

50 M. Fogelholm, "Physical Activity, Fitness and Fatness: Relations to Mortality, Morbidity and Disease Risk Factors. A Systematic Review," *Obesity Reviews* 11, no. 3 (March 2010): 202–21, www.doi.org/10.1111/j.1467-789X.2009.00653.x.

Chapter 3

1 Centar za Mindfulness IDIS, "The History of MBSR and Science behind Mindfulness - Short Video," May 22, 2017, www.youtube.com/watch?v=JJDwgq1kNl0.

2 J. Yu, P. Song, Y. Zhang, and Z. Wei, "Effects of Mindfulness-Based Intervention on the Treatment of Problematic Eating Behaviors: A Systematic Review," *Journal of Alternative and Complementary Medicine* 26, no. 8 (August 2020): 666–79, www.doi.org/10.1089/acm.2019.0163.

3 E. Robinson, P. Aveyard, A. Daley, K. Jolly, A. Lewis, D. Lycett, and S. Higgs, "Eating Attentively: A Systematic Review and Meta-Analysis of the Effect of Food Intake Memory and Awareness on Eating," *American Journal of Clinical Nutrition* 97, no. 4 (2013): 728–42, www.doi.org/10.3945/ajcn.112.045245.

4 B. K. Hölzel, J. Carmody, M. Vangel, C. Congleton, S. M. Yerramsetti, T. Gard, and S. W. Lazar, "Mindfulness Practice Leads to Increases in Regional Brain Gray Matter Density," *Psychiatry Research: Neuroimaging* 191, no. 1 (2011): 36–43, www.doi.org/10.1016/j.pscychresns.2010.08.006.

5 K. C. Fox, S. Nijeboer, M. L. Dixon, J. L. Floman, M. Ellamil, S. P. Rumak, P. Sedlmeier, and K. Christoff, "Is Meditation Associated with Altered Brain Structure? A Systematic Review and Meta-Analysis of Morphometric Neuroimaging in Meditation Practitioners," *Neuroscience and Biobehavioral Review* 43 (June 2014): 48–73, www.doi.org/10.1016/j.neubiorev.2014.03.016.

6 C. Congleton, B. Hölzel, and S. Lazar, "Mindfulness Can Literally Change Your Brain," *Harvard Business Review*, January 8, 2015, www.hbr.org/2015/01/mindfulness-can-literally-change-your-brain.

7 "Jon Kabat-Zinn: Defining Mindfulness," Mindful, January 11, 2017, www.mindful.org/jon-kabat-zinn-defining-mindfulness/.

8 Jon Kabat-Zinn, *Full Catastrophe Living: Using the Wisdom of Your Body and Mind to Face Stress, Pain, and Illness* (New York: Bantam Books, 2013), 7.

9 B. Gardner, P. Lally, and J. Wardle, "Making Health Habitual: The Psychology of 'Habit-Formation' and General Practice," *British Journal of General Practice* 62, no. 605 (2012): 664–66, www.doi.org/10.3399/bjgp12X659466; Tara Parker-Pope, "How to Build Healthy Habits," *New York Times*, February 18, 2020, www.nytimes.com/2020/02/18/well/mind/how-to-build-healthy-habits.html.

10 P. Lally, C. H. M. van Jaarsveld, H. W. W. Potts, and J. Wardle, "How Are Habits Formed: Modelling Habit Formation in the Real World," *European Journal of Social Psychology* 40, no. 6 (2010): 998–1009, www.doi.org/10.1002/ejsp.674.

11 Jon Kabat-Zinn, *Falling Awake: How to Practice Mindfulness in Everyday Life* (New York: Hachette Books, 2018).

Chapter 4

1 B. F. Skinner, *Science and Human Behavior* (New York: Macmillan, 1953).

2 M. E. P. Seligman, "Learned Helplessness," *Annual Review of Medicine* 23, no. 1 (1972): 407–12, www.doi.org/10.1146/annurev.me.23.020172.002203.

3 Elizabeth Scott, "The Toxic Effects of Negative Self-Talk," Verywell Mind, February 25, 2020, www.verywellmind.com/negative-self-talk-and-how-it-affects-us -4161304.

4 Kerry S. O'Brien, Janet D. Latner, Rebecca M. Puhl, Lenny R. Vartanian, Claudia Giles, Konstadina Griva, and Adrian Carter, "The Relationship between Weight Stigma and Eating Behavior Is Explained by Weight Bias Internalization and Psychological Distress," *Appetite* 102 (2016): 70–76, www.doi.org/10.1016/j.appet .2016.02.032; Rachel D. Marshall, Janet D. Latner, and Akihiko Masuda, "Internalized Weight Bias and Disordered Eating: The Mediating Role of Body Image Avoidance and Drive for Thinness," *Frontiers in Psychology* 10 (January 22, 2020): 2999, www.doi.org/10.3389/fpsyg.2019.02999; Natasha A. Schvey and Marney A. White, "The Internalization of Weight Bias Is Associated with Severe Eating Pathology among Lean Individuals," *Eating Behaviors* 17 (April 2015): 1–5, www.doi.org /10.1016/j.eatbeh.2014.11.001.

5 Annette Kämmerer, "The Scientific Underpinnings and Impacts of Shame," *Scientific American*, August 9, 2019, www.scientificamerican.com/article/the-scientific -underpinnings-and-impacts-of-shame/.

6 Kristin Neff, "Definition and Three Elements of Self-Compassion," Self-Compassion, July 9, 2020, www.self-compassion.org/the-three-elements-of-self-compassion-2/.

7 Kristin Neff, Stephanie Rude, and Kristin Kirkpatrick, "An Examination of Self-Compassion in Relation to Positive Psychological Functioning and Personality Traits," *Journal of Research in Personality* 41, no. 4 (2007): 908–16, www.doi.org /10.1016/j.jrp.2006.08.002; Emma Seppala, "The Scientific Benefits of Self-Compassion," Center for Compassion and Altruism Research and Education, June 28, 2017, http://ccare.stanford.edu/uncategorized/the-scientific-benefits-of-self -compassion-infographic/.

8 Alberto Voci, Chiara Veneziani, and Giulia Fuochi, "Relating Mindfulness, Heartfulness, and Psychological Well-Being: The Role of Self-Compassion and Gratitude," *Mindfulness* 10, no. 2 (2019): 339–51, www.doi.org/10.1007/s12671-018-0978-0.

9 E. R. Albertson, K. D. Neff, and K. E. Dill-Shackleford, "Self-Compassion and Body Dissatisfaction in Women: A Randomized Controlled Trial of a Brief Meditation Intervention," *Mindfulness* 6, no. 3 (2015): 444–54, www.doi.org/10.1007 /s12671-014-0277-3.

10 Kristin Neff, "Self-Appreciation: The Flip Side of Self-Compassion," Self-Compassion, February 21, 2015, www.self-compassion.org/self-appreciation-the-flip-side-of -self-compassion/.

11 Alberto Voci, Chiara Veneziani, and Giulia Fuochi, "Relating Mindfulness, Heart-fulness, and Psychological Well-Being: The Role of Self-Compassion and Gratitude," *Mindfulness* 10, no. 2 (2019): 339–51, www.doi.org/10.1007/s12671-018-0978-0.

12 J. Dunaev, C. Markey, and P. Brochu, "An Attitude of Gratitude: The Effects of Body-Focused Gratitude on Weight Bias Internalization and Body Image," *Body Image* 25 (2018): 9–13, www.doi.org/10.1016/j.bodyim.2018.01.006.

13 P. K. Kohler, L. E. Manhart, and W. E. Lafferty, "Abstinence-Only and Comprehensive Sex Education and the Initiation of Sexual Activity and Teen Pregnancy," *Journal of Adolescent Health* 42, no. 4 (2008): 344–51, www.doi.org/10.1016/j.jadohealth.2007.08.026.

14 J. Dunaev, C. Markey, and P. Brochu, "An Attitude of Gratitude: The Effects of Body-Focused Gratitude on Weight Bias Internalization and Body Image," *Body Image* 25 (2018): 9–13, www.doi.org/10.1016/j.bodyim.2018.01.006.

Chapter 6

1 J. Steen, "We Found Out If It Really Takes 20 Minutes to Feel Full," Huffington Post, November 10, 2016, www.huffingtonpost.com.au/2016/11/09/we-found-out-if-it-really-takes-20-minutes-to-feel-full_a_21602736/.

2 C. K. Miller, J. L. Kristeller, A. Headings, and H. Nagaraja, "Comparison of a Mindful Eating Intervention to a Diabetes Self-Management Intervention among Adults with Type 2 Diabetes: A Randomized Controlled Trial," *Health Education and Behavior* 41, no. 2 (2014): 145–54, www.doi.org/10.1177/1090198113493092.

3 Charles Piller, "Dubious Diagnosis: The War on 'Prediabetes' Could Be a Boon for Pharma—but Is It Good Medicine?" *Science*, March 7, 2019, www.sciencemag.org/news/2019/03/war-prediabetes-could-be-boon-pharma-it-good-medicine.

4 "Why People Become Overweight," Harvard Health Publishing, Harvard Medical School, June 2009, updated June 2019, www.health.harvard.edu/staying-healthy/why-people-become-overweight.

Chapter 7

1 G. Cook, "How the Sense of Taste Has Shaped Who We Are," *Scientific American*, January 13, 2015, www.scientificamerican.com/article/how-the-sense-of-taste-has-shaped-who-we-are/.

2 Y. P. Zverev, "Effects of Caloric Deprivation and Satiety on Sensitivity of the Gustatory System," *BMC Neuroscience* 5 (2004): 5, www.doi.org/10.1186/1471-2202-5-5.

3 O. Fu, Y. Iwai, M. Narukawa, A. W. Ishikawa, K. K. Ishii, K. Murata, Y. Yoshimura, K. Touhara, T. Misaka, Y. Minokoshi, and K. Nakajima, "Hypothalamic Neuronal Circuits Regulating Hunger-Induced Taste Modification," *Nature Communications* 10 (2019): 4560, www.doi.org/10.1038/s41467-019-12478-x.

4 Carol Lawson, "Julia Child Boiling, Answers Her Critics," *New York Times*, June 20, 1990, www.nytimes.com/1990/06/20/garden/julia-child-boiling-answers-her-critics.html.

5 G. Cook, "How the Sense of Taste Has Shaped Who We Are," *Scientific American*, January 13, 2015, www.scientificamerican.com/article/how-the-sense-of-taste -has-shaped-who-we-are/.

6 A. L. Huang, X. Chen, M. A. Hoon, J. Chandrashekar, W. Guo, D. Tränkner, N. J. Ryba, and C. S. Zuker, "The Cells and Logic for Mammalian Sour Taste Detection," *Nature* 442, no. 7105 (August 24, 2006): 934–38, www.doi.org/10.1038 /nature05084.

7 K. Sato, S. Endo, and H. Tomita. "Sensitivity of Three Loci on the Tongue and Soft Palate to Four Basic Tastes in Smokers and Non-Smokers," *Acta Oto-Laryngologica* 122, no. 4 (2002): 74–82, www.doi.org/10.1080/00016480260046445; A. O'Connor, "The Claim: Tongue Is Mapped into Four Areas of Taste," *New York Times*, November 10, 2008, www.nytimes.com/2008/11/11/health/11real.html.

8 B. R. Carruth, P. J. Ziegler, A. Gordon, S. I. Barr, "Prevalence of Picky Eaters among Infants and Toddlers and Their Caregivers' Decisions about Offering a New Food," *Journal of the American Dietetic Association* 104, suppl. 1 (January 2004): S57–64, www.doi.org/10.1016/j.jada.2003.10.024.

9 J. A. Mennella, C. P. Jagnow, and G. K. Beauchamp, "Prenatal and Postnatal Flavor Learning by Human Infants," *Pediatrics* 107, no. 6 (2001): E88, www.doi.org /10.1542/peds.107.6.e88.

10 L. Hallberg, E. Björn-Rasmussen, L. Rossander, and R. Suwanik, "Iron Absorption from Southeast Asian Diets. II. Role of Various Factors That Might Explain Low Absorption," *American Journal of Clinical Nutrition* 30, no. 4 (April 1977): 539–48, www.doi.org/10.1093/ajcn/30.4.539.

11 H. Brown, "Go with Your Gut," *New York Times*, February 20, 2006, www.nytimes .com/2006/02/20/opinion/go-with-your-gut.html.

12 J. J. Arch, K. W. Brown, R. J. Goodman, M. D. Della Porta, L. J. Kiken, and S. Tillman, "Enjoying Food without Caloric Cost: The Impact of Brief Mindfulness on Laboratory Eating Outcomes," *Behaviour Research and Therapy* 79 (2016): 23–34, www.doi.org/10.1016/j.brat.2016.02.002.

13 B. Khoury, T. Lecomte, G. Fortin, M. Masse, P. Therien, V. Bouchard, M. A. Chapleau, K. Paquin, and S. G. Hofmann, "Mindfulness-Based Therapy: A Comprehensive Meta-Analysis," *Clinical Psychology Review* 33, no. 6 (August 2013): 763–71, www.doi.org/10.1016/j.cpr.2013.05.005.

Chapter 8

1 G. A. Soliman, "Dietary Cholesterol and the Lack of Evidence in Cardiovascular Disease," *Nutrients* 10, no. 6 (2018): 780, www.doi.org/10.3390/nu10060780.

2 Andrew Jacobs, "Scientific Panel on New Dietary Guidelines Draws Criticism from Health Advocates," *New York Times*, June 17, 2020, www.nytimes.com/2020/06/17 /health/diet-nutrition-guidelines.html.

3 John C. Peters, Holly R. Wyatt, Gary D. Foster, Zhaoxing Pan, Alexis C. Wojtanowski, Stephanie S. Vander Veur, Sharon J. Herring, Carrie Brill, and James O. Hill, "The Effects of Water and Non-nutritive Sweetened Beverages on Weight Loss during a 12-Week Weight Loss Treatment Program," *Obesity* 22, no. 6 (June 2014): 1415–21, www.doi.org/10.1002/oby.20737.

4 Ahmed O'Connor, "Coca-Cola Funds Scientists Who Shift Blame for Obesity Away from Bad Diets," *New York Times*, August 9, 2015, https://well.blogs.nytimes .com/2015/08/09/coca-cola-funds-scientists-who-shift-blame-for-obesity-away-from -bad-diets/.

5 A. Sifferlin, "Big Soda-Funded Studies Don't Often Link Drinks to Obesity," *Time*, November 1, 2016, www.time.com/4553110/soda-industry-sugar-obesity-diabetes/.

6 Marion Nestle, "Food Industry Funding of Nutrition Research: The Relevance of History for Current Debates," *JAMA Internal Medicine* 176, no. 11 (2016): 1685–86, www.doi.org/10.1001/jamainternmed.2016.5400.

7 Candida J. Rebello, Yi-Fang Chu, William D. Johnson, Corby K. Martin, Hongmei Han, Nicolas Bordenave, Yuhui Shi, Marianne O'Shea, and Frank L. Greenway, "The Role of Meal Viscosity and Oat B-Glucan Characteristics in Human Appetite Control: A Randomized Crossover Trial," *Nutrition Journal* 13, no. 49 (2014), www.doi .org/10.1186/1475-2891-13-49; Candice Choi, "AP Exclusive: How Candy Makers Shape Nutrition Science," Associated Press, June 2, 2016, www.apnews.com/article /f9483d554430445fa6566bb0aaa293d1.

8 David L. Katz, Anna Davidhi, Yingying Ma, Yasemin Kavak, Lauren Bifulco, and Valentine Yanchou Njike, "Effects of Walnuts on Endothelial Function in Overweight Adults with Visceral Obesity: A Randomized, Controlled, Crossover Trial," *Journal of the American College of Nutrition* 31, no. 6 (2012): 415–23, www.doi.org /10.1080/07315724.2012.10720468; Valentine Yanchou Njike, Rockiy Ayettey, Paul Petraro, Judith A. Treu, and David L. Katz, "Walnut Ingestion in Adults at Risk for Diabetes: Effects on Body Composition, Diet Quality, and Cardiac Risk Measures," *BMJ Open Diabetes Research and Care* 3, no. 1 (2015): 3, www.doi.org/10.1136 /bmjdrc-2015-000115.

9 Daniel J. Lamport, Clare L. Lawton, Natasha Merat, Hamish Jamson, Kyriaki Myrissa, Denise Hofman, Helen K. Chadwick, Frits Quadt, JoLynne D. Wightman, and Louise Dye, "Concord Grape Juice, Cognitive Function, and Driving Performance: A 12-Week, Placebo-Controlled, Randomized Crossover Trial in Mothers of Preteen Children," *American Journal of Clinical Nutrition* 103, no. 3 (March 2016): 775–83, www.doi.org/10.3945/ajcn.115.114553; Julia Belluz, "Nutrition Research Is Deeply Biased by Food Companies: A New Book Explains Why," Vox, October 31,

2018, www.vox.com/2018/10/31/18037756/superfoods-food-science-marion
-nestle-book.

10 L. I. Lesser, C. B. Ebbeling, M. Goozner, D. Wypij, and D. S. Ludwig, "Relationship
between Funding Source and Conclusion among Nutrition-Related Scientific Articles,"
PLoS Medicine 4, no. 1 (2007): e5, www.doi.org/10.1371/journal.pmed.0040005.

11 Marion Nestle, "Six Industry-Funded Studies. The Score for the Year: 156/12," Food
Politics, March 18, 2006, www.foodpolitics.com/2016/03/six-industry-funded
-studies-the-score-for-the-year-15612/.

12 A. J. Hill, "The Psychology of Food Craving," *Proceedings of the Nutrition Society* 66,
no. 2 (May 2007): 277–85, www.doi.org/10.1017/S0029665107005502.

13 J. M. Hormes and M. A. Niemiec, "Does Culture Create Craving? Evidence from
the Case of Menstrual Chocolate Craving," *PLoS One* 12, no. 7 (2017): e0181445,
www.doi.org/10.1371/journal.pone.0181445.

14 K. Sheikh, "How Gut Bacteria Tell Their Hosts What to Eat," *Scientific American*,
April 25, 2017, www.scientificamerican.com/article/how-gut-bacteria-tell-their-hosts
-what-to-eat/; C. Zimmer, "Our Microbiome May Be Looking Out for Itself," *New
York Times*, August 14, 2014, www.nytimes.com/2014/08/14/science/our
-microbiome-may-be-looking-out-for-itself.html.

15 R. Leitão-Gonçalves, Z. Carvalho-Santos, A. P. Francisco, G. T. Fioreze, M. Anjos,
C. Baltazar, A. P. Elias, P. M. Itskov, M. D. W. Piper, and C. Ribeiro, "Commensal
Bacteria and Essential Amino Acids Control Food Choice Behavior and Reproduc-
tion," *PLoS Biology* 15, no. 4 (2017): e2000862, www.doi.org/10.1371/journal
.pbio.2000862; S. Love, "Are Gut Bacteria Driving Your Cravings?" Vice, April 25,
2017, www.vice.com/en/article/nzpqwq/are-gut-bacteria-driving-your-cravings.

16 F. A. Duca, T. D. Swartz, Y. Sakar, and M. Covasa, "Increased Oral Detection, but
Decreased Intestinal Signaling for Fats in Mice Lacking Gut Microbiota," *PLoS One*
7, no. 6 (2012): e39748, www.doi.org/10.1371/journal.pone.0039748; J. Alcock, C.
C. Maley, and C. A. Aktipis, "Is Eating Behavior Manipulated by the Gastrointestinal
Microbiota? Evolutionary Pressures and Potential Mechanisms," *BioEssays* 36, no. 10
(2014): 940–49, www.doi.org/10.1002/bies.201400071.

17 J. Alcock, C. C. Maley, and C. A. Aktipis, "Is Eating Behavior Manipulated by the
Gastrointestinal Microbiota? Evolutionary Pressures and Potential Mechanisms,"
BioEssays 36, no. 10 (2014): 940–49, www.doi.org/10.1002/bies.201400071.

18 M. L. Pelchat and S. Schaefer, "Dietary Monotony and Food Cravings in Young
and Elderly Adults, *Physiology and Behavior* 68, no. 3 (January 2000): 353–59,
www.doi.org/10.1016/s0031-9384(99)00190-0.

19 Kristen Bruinsma and Douglas L. Taren, "Chocolate: Food or Drug?" *Journal of
American Dietetic Association* 99, no. 10 (1999): 1249–56, www.doi.org/10.1016
/S0002-8223(99)00307-7.

20 Eric G. Krause, Annette D. de Kloet, Jonathan N. Flak, Michael D. Smeltzer, Matia
B. Solomon, Nathan K. Evanson, Stephen C. Woods, Randall R. Sakai, and James

P. Herman, "Hydration State Controls Stress Responsiveness and Social Behavior," *Journal of Neuroscience* 31, no. 4 (2011): 5470–76, www.doi.org/10.1523 /JNEUROSCI.6078-10.2011.

Chapter 9

1 L. Nummenmaa, E. Glerean, R. Hari, and J. Hietanen, "Bodily Maps of Emotions," *Proceedings of the National Academy of Sciences* 111, no. 2 (2014): 646–51, www.doi .org/10.1073/pnas.1321664111.

Chapter 10

1 V. E. Frankl, *Man's Search for Meaning: An Introduction to Logotherapy* (New York: Simon & Schuster, 1984).

2 S. Freud, *Civilization and Its Discontents* (New York: W. W. Norton, 1964).

3 A. H. Maslow, "A Theory of Human Motivation," *Psychological Review* 50, no. 4 (1943): 370–96, www.doi.org/10.1037/h0054346.

4 C. B. Becker, K. Middlemass, B. Taylor, C. Johnson, and F. Gomez, "Food Insecurity and Eating Disorder Pathology," *International Journal of Eating Disorders* 50, no. 9 (September 2017): 1031–40, www.doi.org/10.1002/eat.22735.

5 A. R. Hochschild and A. Machung, *The Second Shift: Working Parents and the Revolution at Home* (New York: Viking, 1989).

6 "Audre Lorde," Poetry Foundation, n.d., retrieved December 13, 2020, www .poetryfoundation.org/poets/Audre-lorde; Audre Lorde, *A Burst of Light: Essays* (Ithaca, NY: Firebrand Books, 1988), 130.

7 Barbara Riegel and Debra K. Moser, "Self-Care: An Update on the State of the Science One Decade Later," *Journal of Cardiovascular Nursing* 33, no. 5 (2018): 404–07, www.doi.org/10.1097/JCN.0000000000000517.

8 "Get the Facts: Drinking Water and Intake," Centers for Disease Control and Prevention, August 9, 2016, www.cdc.gov/nutrition/data-statistics/plain-water-the-healthier -choice.html; T. Newman, "The 7 Wonders of Poop," *Medical News Today*, February 1, 2019, www.medicalnewstoday.com/articles/324254.

9 K. Zelman, "The Wonders of Water," WebMD, January 14, 2010, www.webmd.com /a-to-z-guides/features/wonders-of-water.

10 "How Much Sleep Do I Need?" Centers for Disease Control and Prevention, March 2, 2017, www.cdc.gov/sleep/about_sleep/how_much_sleep.html; "How Much Sleep Do We Really Need?" National Sleep Foundation, October 9, 2020, www.sleepfoundation .org/articles/how-much-sleep-do-we-really-need.

11 "Sleep Home Page—Sleep and Sleep Disorders," Centers for Disease Control and Prevention, April 15, 2020, www.cdc.gov/sleep/index.html.

12 "Why Sleep Is Important," American Psychological Association, n.d., retrieved October 18, 2020, www.apa.org/topics/sleep/why.

13 "Why Sleep Is Important," American Psychological Association, n.d., retrieved October 18, 2020, www.apa.org/topics/sleep/why.

14 "Sleep Home Page—Sleep and Sleep Disorders," Centers for Disease Control and Prevention, April 15, 2020, www.cdc.gov/sleep/index.html.

15 "More Sleep Would Make Us Happier, Healthier and Safer," American Psychological Association, February 2014, www.apa.org/action/resources/research-in-action /sleep-deprivation.

16 L. Brits, "The Importance of Making Time for Leisure," Medium, October 11, 2019, www.medium.com/live-your-life-on-purpose/the-importance-of-making-time-for -leisure-33d6cf3788e0.

17 J. Holt-Lunstad, T. B. Smith, M. Baker, T. Harris, and D. Stephenson, "Loneliness and Social Isolation as Risk Factors for Mortality: A Meta-Analytic Review," *Perspectives on Psychological Science* 10, no. 2 (2015): 227–37, www.doi.org/10.1177 /1745691614568352.

18 A. Novotney, "The Risks of Social Isolation," *Monitor on Psychology* 50, no. 5 (March 2020), www.apa.org/monitor/2019/05/ce-corner-isolation.

19 D. Umberson and J. K. Montez, "Social Relationships and Health: A Flashpoint for Health Policy," *Journal of Health and Social Behavior* 51, no. S1 (2010): S54–66, www.doi.org/10.1177/0022146510383501.

20 C. Reissman, A. Aron, and M. R. Bergen, "Shared Activities and Marital Satisfaction: Causal Direction and Self-Expansion versus Boredom," *Journal of Social and Personal Relationships* 10, no. 2 (1993): 243–54, www.doi.org/10.1177/026540759301000205.

21 Tenga Co. Ltd., "World's Largest Masturbation Survey Uncovers How Traditional Views of Masculinity Prevent Men from Having Fulfilling Sex Lives and Relationships," June 27, 2018, www.prnewswire.com/news-releases/worlds-largest -masturbation-survey-uncovers-how-traditional-views-of-masculinity-prevent -men-from-having-fulfilling-sex-lives--relationships-300638644.html.

22 J. L. Shulman and S. G. Horne, "The Use of Self-Pleasure: Masturbation and Body Image among African American and European American Women," *Psychology of Women Quarterly* 27, no. 3 (2003): 262–69, www.doi.org/10.1111/1471-6402 .00106; Y. Pujols, B. N. Seal, and C. M. Meston, "The Association between Sexual Satisfaction and Body Image in Women," *Journal of Sexual Medicine* 7, no. 2 (2010): 905–16, www.doi.org/10.1111/j.1743-6109.2009.01604.x.

23 M. Reece, D. Herbenick, V. Schick, S. Sanders, B. Dodge, and J. D. Fortenberry, "Sexual Behaviors in the US" (presented at Sexual Health Across the Lifespan: Practical Applications, Colorado Department of Public Health and Environment, Denver, CO, 2013).

24 Tenga Co. Ltd., "World's Largest Masturbation Survey Uncovers How Traditional Views of Masculinity Prevent Men from Having Fulfilling Sex Lives and Relationships," June 27, 2018, www.prnewswire.com/news-releases/worlds-largest -masturbation-survey-uncovers-how-traditional-views-of-masculinity-prevent-men -from-having-fulfilling-sex-lives--relationships-300638644.html.

25 D. Herbenick, T.-C. (J.) Fu, J. Arter, S. A. Sanders, and B. Dodge, "Women's Experiences with Genital Touching, Sexual Pleasure, and Orgasm: Results from a U.S. Probability Sample of Women Ages 18 to 94," *Journal of Sex & Marital Therapy* 44, no. 2 (2018): 201–12, www.doi.org/10.1080/0092623X.2017.1346530.

26 "The 2019 Year in Review," Pornhub, December 11, 2019, www.pornhub.com /insights/2019-year-in-review; A. Cadenet, "More Women Watch (and Enjoy) Porn Than You Ever Realized: A Marie Claire Study," *Marie Claire*, March 29, 2018, www.marieclaire.com/sex-love/a16474/women-porn-habits-study/.

Index

Acknowledgments

This book has been nearly a decade in the making. When I started working on the proposal for it, there were almost no books on mindful eating written from a Health at Every Size (HAES)–informed weight-inclusive perspective. The anti-diet movement has exploded since then, and I feel fortunate to have grown and evolved along with it. This book is very different than the one I would've written ten years ago thanks to what I've learned from others. I'm especially grateful to the HAES community and the fat activists who laid the foundation for this work. While body positivity has surged in popularity over the past several years thanks to social media, the movement wouldn't exist if not for the radical early work of the fat acceptance movement.

To all of my clients who have trusted me to bear witness to your journey and to share your pain, allowing me into your inner world, I feel deeply grateful for the privilege of being your therapist. Your courage, bravery, and resiliency inspire me.

This book wouldn't have happened if not for my agent, Tina Wainscott, and her team at The Seymour Agency. I had all but given up hope that my book-writing dreams would come true when Tina called me out of the blue to ask if I would be interested in working with her. It was like the stars finally aligned! I became pregnant with my younger daughter mere months after signing with the agency, but we (slowly) worked our way through and signed with North Atlantic Books on my daughter's first birthday. I couldn't have asked for a better publishing home than North Atlantic Books. After being told over and over again by others in the publishing world that I can't write a book telling people it's okay to be fat, it was refreshing to work with a publisher that embraced fat acceptance. I'm thankful to the entire team at North Atlantic Books, especially my editor, Shayna Keyles, who guided me through the writing process with support, insight, and kindness; as well as Janelle Ludowise who ushered my book through the final stages of publishing, Julia Sadowski and Bevin Donahue for their help with publicity and marketing, and the team at Penguin Random House for distribution. Writing a book is an incredibly vulnerable process, and I am grateful to have been met with warmth and compassion at North Atlantic Books.

I would be lost without my professional community of therapists, researchers, eating disorder professionals, and the HAES community. I am grateful for the time and insight of Joy Cox, PhD, and Lindley Ashline, who read an early draft of this book and provided invaluable guidance in making the book more inclusive and accessible. Thank you to Shira Rosenbluth, LCSW, for being my sounding board, helping me build my platform online, unpacking ideas with me, and showing me what true activism looks like. Jenna Hollenstein, RDN, has been an unwavering source of support, both in the book-writing process and in life. The seeds for this proposal were planted with Sandra Feinblum, LCSW. We didn't make it to the publishing finishing line together, but I value your early input and especially the time we spent together in that process. Thank you to Stephen Snyder, MD, for generously spending the time to review my proposal and provide guidance and encouragement throughout the publishing process. The International Association of Eating Disorders Professionals New York Chapter community has kept me from feeling alone in the isolation that can be private practice. The peer supervision groups I participate in have served a similar purpose and helped me think deeper about my clinical work. The Center for Mindful Eating has grounded me in mindfulness and connected me with other practitioners dedicated to returning mindful eating to its weight-inclusive core. I am grateful to the "obesity" research and bariatric-surgery community that welcomed me in, trained me, and taught me so much (including just how much we *don't* know!). I value the relationships forged through many years of working and conferencing together. The Health at Every Size Therapists and Nutritionists group on Facebook has been an invaluable resource in deepening my thinking about HAES. I'm so grateful to all who put labor into responding to questions and posts, provided article recommendations, and reminded me that, even though at times it can feel like we are the only ones going against the weight-normative tide, we are far from alone.

My friends have been incredible sources of support and guidance in this project. I am grateful for every conversation we had about this bumpy road of writing, publishing, and branding. I especially want to thank all of my friends (and friends of friends) who made introductions to agents, publishers, and editors and helped me learn the ropes of the publishing industry. When I first had the idea to write a book, I had no clue what was involved. Your guidance was vital, and I am grateful for the time and energy you dedicated to this project.

I couldn't ask for a better partner than my husband, Greg. He is my biggest cheerleader and encouraged me to keep moving forward, even when I doubted myself. During the writing process, he took on more than his fair share of childcare and household responsibilities (sometimes entertaining the kids on his own for entire weekends—all in the midst of a global pandemic—and doing the cooking and cleaning to boot!). He also helped with some of the medical details in the book, especially surrounding diabetes and metabolism. I'm eternally grateful for his insight, support, and love.

I wouldn't have been able to write this book without our nanny, Tasha. She's been in our lives since our kids were born, and I trust her completely with their care—that is a rare gift that provided me with the time and focus I needed to write this book. My appreciation is beyond words.

I'm grateful to my mother, who planted the writing seed many years ago with her unbridled enthusiasm for books, words, and writing. She has zealously praised my achievements throughout my life, and this book is no different; I appreciate all the encouragement she has provided.

My in-laws, Herb, Shelli, and Aly, have been my tireless champions, checking in on my progress with the book, even during the years that very little progress had been made. I'm grateful to my sister, Laurie, and niece Liz, for all their support in life; you both know how much you mean to me. My cousin Janet, who was taken from us too soon, was an inspiration in her tireless fight for the rights of women across the world, and I'm grateful for the wisdom she shared with me in the early stages of my proposal.

My daughters, Roberta and Emilia, are my inspiration. I pray that we can raise this generation of girls without the body shame that plagued my generation and the generations before me.

Every milestone reminds me of the loss of my dad, over eight years ago now, who I miss every day. I know that if he were here, he would be proud as could be, telling everyone he knows about this accomplishment. It is a gift to have someone in your life who truly believes in you; if I can be even a fraction of how great he thought I was, I will have succeeded.

About the Author

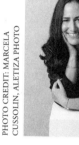

ALEXIS CONASON, PsyD, CEDS-S, is a clinical psychologist and eating disorder specialist in private practice in New York City. She is the founder of The Anti-Diet Plan, a weight-inclusive online mindful eating program. She was previously a research associate at the New York Nutrition Obesity Research Center in affiliation with Columbia University. Her research has been published in peer-reviewed journals, she is a frequent speaker at conferences, and she has been featured widely as an expert on the topics of mindful eating, body image, and diet culture in the media. You can find her on social media @theantidietplan.

A lifelong New Yorker, Conason lives in Manhattan with her husband and two daughters. She loves all things related to food including cooking, food shopping, watching food shows on TV, and of course eating! But most rewarding is helping her clients transform their relationship with food and experience the joys of eating. She is a fierce advocate for helping people recognize and question the societal norms that encourage their feeling not good enough about themselves so they can stop fixating on shrinking their bodies and reclaim the space that they deserve in the world.